ORGANISING CARE
AROUND PATIENTS

MANCHESTER
1824

Manchester University Press

ORGANISING CARE AROUND PATIENTS

Stories from the frontline of the NHS

**NAOMI CHAMBERS AND
JEREMY TAYLOR**

Manchester University Press

Published by Manchester University Press
Oxford Road, Manchester M13 9PL

www.manchesteruniversitypress.co.uk

British Library Cataloguing-in-Publication Data
A catalogue record for this book is available from the British Library

ISBN   978 1 5261 4745 5   hardback

ISBN   978 1 5261 4746 2   paperback

First published 2021

Typeset
by New Best-set Typesetters Ltd

CONTENTS

Audio recordings of the testimonies featured in the book are available here: www.manchesteropenhive.com/NHSstories/audio

FIGURES

ACKNOWLEDGEMENTS

We would like to thank the storytellers for their time and for their generosity in sharing their experiences. We are also grateful to Elaine Clark, who has stepped forward to provide an audio version of this book.

⟫ 1 ⟪

INTRODUCTION

The same month that my mum was diagnosed with Alzheimer's and dementia, my employer asked me to relocate down south. I thought, I can't really do that, she's in her hour of need, so I'll take redundancy. That was probably ten or eleven years ago now. I was 42 then. She didn't want to go in a care home, so I said, I'll do as much as I can to prevent that. When she was diagnosed, I was disappointed with the service she got from the NHS. It was a case of, right, there's your diagnosis, you've got mixed dementia, Alzheimer's and vascular dementia, here's some tablets, come back in twelve months, and that's it. This is a massive, life-changing thing for her and for her family. We didn't know what to expect. (**James**, in Chapter 7)

SECTION 1   INTRODUCTION

Ill health is a burden. For many of us, when it comes, it is a passing inconvenience and the burden is light. But ill health can also come as a devastating bolt from the blue, like a stroke or cancer or COVID-19, or as a life-defining or life-limiting chronic condition. At its worst, the experience of ill health is measured out in pain, fear, anxiety, depression, exhaustion, confusion and much more besides.

No healthcare system can eliminate these bad experiences, which are inherent features of illness. Nor can it remove the intrusiveness of treatment and procedures: the worry of tests, the pain of surgery, the hassle of getting to the hospital, the side effects of medications, the labour of caring for loved ones. But healthcare can do much to make the experiences better, or worse.

In its millions of daily encounters with patients and their families, the NHS saves lives, relieves suffering and helps people manage, on a massive scale. But it also creates bad experiences. Patients wait too long, struggle to get information and wear themselves out navigating bureaucracy. Their medical notes get lost, the different professionals looking after them don't talk to each other, and sometimes it feels as though no one is taking responsibility. Countless acts of kindness and compassion are offset by the occasions when staff are impatient, dismissive, high-handed or worse. Massive reorganising designed for the general good – such as the changes the NHS had to make during the COVID-19 pandemic – might have a devastating impact on individuals. Not all care is safe and sometimes it causes harm.

Why this book?

The NHS has long declared its commitment to "patient-centred care", but a large gap remains between the fine words and the reality. Care often feels as if it is designed for the convenience of the organisations that deliver it, and not enough around patients and their families, or even around the frontline staff who provide it. Why does this happen? What does it feel like? And, most importantly, what can be done about it?

This book aims to stimulate reflection on these questions by listening closely to those at the frontline. It provides accounts from patients, carers and healthcare professionals who are patients about what it's like when services get it right and wrong, from birth up to the end of life. Quite simply, we want to draw on the power of storytelling – increasingly valued as a tool for learning – to help practitioners understand how to deliver better care.

There is a growing literature of first-person accounts both from patients and from healthcare professionals. This book differs by providing a collection of narratives, from a variety of viewpoints and stages in life, to paint a rich and varied picture. Alongside these narratives we provide some context: an overview of the history, theory and evidential underpinnings of moves towards a more patient-centred approach to care. We present some of the theory and practice of storytelling in the context of healthcare. And we seek to help the reader to draw out the practical learnings from the individual accounts.

This book is primarily focussed on England. Our storytellers relate experiences of the NHS in England, and our policy and historical scene-setting is also mostly from an English perspective. The English healthcare system is by far the largest in the UK and one of the largest among high-income countries. It is grappling with problems, many of which are global in nature, such as the need to adapt healthcare to the growing populations of people with multiple long-term conditions. We are confident therefore that the themes and learnings that we draw out in the book, while reflecting English particularities, will also have broader resonance.

Who is this book for?

This book is aimed primarily at undergraduate, postgraduate and research students in the healthcare professions, and students and scholars interested in management, health and social policy, and leadership. We believe it will also be of interest to policymakers, NHS managers, healthcare professionals, the voluntary sector operating in the health space, and a broader reading public who care about the NHS and want to understand it better.

How to read this book

This introductory chapter sets the scene and is structured as follows. Section 2 explains what we mean by organising care around patients and our alternative term "patient-centred care". We set out the key characteristics of patient-centred care and explain why it is important. Section 3 provides a brief history of developments in patient-centred care, in policy, attitudes and practice. Section 4 reviews, in light of this history, whether and to what extent the NHS can be viewed as patient-centred and the obstacles to further progress in this direction. Section 5 explains our approach to storytelling as a means of eliciting important truths about patient-centred care. It explains how we found the storytellers, the ethical and methodological issues we encountered, and what we learned from the process of listening to the stories. Finally, Section 6 summarises the structure of the rest of the book and suggests how the reader might engage with and learn from the stories it contains.

SECTION 2   ORGANISING CARE AROUND PATIENTS: WHAT IS IT AND WHY DOES IT MATTER?

"Organising care around patients" is not a technical term, nor is it a single thing. We think of it as a family of attitudes, practices and behaviours. Here are some of the ways it is most commonly framed:

- **Understanding and valuing what matters to patients** (and doing something about it). This is exemplified by the NHS commitment to measuring key domains of patient experience, such as access to care, physical comfort and emotional support, as described in the NHS Patient Experience Framework (Department of Health, 2011).
- **Seeing the whole person**. The approach often described as person-centred has been well-summarised by the think tank the Health Foundation as care which treats people with dignity, compassion and respect and which is personalised, coordinated and empowering (Health Foundation, 2016). It is an approach often contrasted with the all-too-common experience of being seen as a "case", disease or body part and finding oneself battling powerlessly against a technocratic and bureaucratic system. It is an approach which also values the relational as well as the technical aspects of care: listening to the patient, treating them as a person, being kind and compassionate. It values "what matters to you?" as much as "what's the matter with you?"
- **Respecting people's rights and autonomy**. This ensures that they have as much choice, voice and control as possible in decisions about their own care – and that of their loved ones – and in what happens more generally in their health services, as a matter of right. A rights-based approach also prioritises equality, diversity and inclusion, opposing discrimination on grounds of race, ethnicity, gender, stigmatised condition or other factors.
- **Being "customer focussed"**. Patients are not the same as shoppers, but there are nonetheless aspects of customer service that patients value and which make a difference to their experience of care (and often also to the safety and effectiveness of the care). These include speed and efficiency, convenience, the availability of meaningful choices, and how well staff relate and communicate. "If only the NHS were better at customer care" is something you often hear when there is a discussion about the difficulties of getting an appointment, of the NHS's outdated attachment to snail mail or of unfriendly receptionists.

Getting the terminology right

These different perspectives on "organising care around patients" overlap to an extent: they are facets of an overall approach that could be summarised as "be kind, be efficient, treat me as a person" and which is often termed patient-centred care. In fact, there is no definitive terminology in this territory, partly reflecting the variety of perspectives and approaches. Thus some commentators prefer "person-centred", objecting to the word "patient" as narrow and demeaning. "Patient" emphasises one's lack of agency and control: as a sick person my role is to wait "patiently" while others do things to me. "Patient" can also be seen to exclude people who are of vital importance to the patient, such as their family, friends and informal carers.

Others prefer "people" to "person" because they want to emphasise the collective: we live in communities which have a powerful impact on our health and which have agency in their own right. Even "centred" is contested by those who think it lacks ambition and who would prefer a "patient-led" NHS. Others will take the view that patient-centredness is something of a distraction when the NHS has a relatively minor impact on health compared with the wider social and economic factors: social class, income, ethnicity, housing and employment, for example. Some activists would rather be working to promote healthier communities than risk being co-opted into tokenistic activities by the box-ticking NHS managers.

It is as well to be aware of these linguistic debates because they indicate where different philosophies of health and care come into conflict with each other. For our purposes, we will stick with "patient-centred" because – for all its semantic drawbacks – it is a sufficiently explanatory and well-understood term in the context of a book about the NHS.

Why is patient-centred care important?

Just as patient-centred care is not a single thing, so there is not a single rationale for it. Rather there are several arguments, reflecting the different perspectives considered above, and which draw upon different kinds of world view, theory or evidence. They partly overlap and together they can be seen as a compelling case for patient-centred care.

- **The moral case**. There is a straightforward moral case for patient-centredness: that it is simply the right thing to do.
- **The clinical case**. This makes the case that patient-centred care leads to better outcomes from healthcare. It cites a body of evidence showing that patients who have agency – who are actively engaged in decisions about their health and care – are more likely to cope well, have a good experience of care and report good outcomes of healthcare.

- **The person-centred case**. This argues for the need to correct the dehumanising and alienating features of modern, science-based healthcare. It stresses the importance to patients of being seen as and treated as a whole person. It argues for holistic, seamless, joined-up care which overcomes professional and organisational silos such as the separate approaches to physical and mental ill health and to health and social care.
- **The justice case**. This makes access to patient-centred care a question of human rights and social justice. It has inspired generations of activists – for example, those who have campaigned for the rights of disabled people and those detained under the Mental Health Act. It sees the more equal distribution of power as fundamental to healthcare and insists on "no decision about me without me". The justice case draws attention to the fact that those with the worst health and the worst outcomes of healthcare are often those with the least voice in decisions that affect both. It insists that a patient-centred approach must also be tailored to the circumstances, needs and preferences of different groups and communities in order to reduce health inequalities and promote greater equality and inclusion.
- **The economic case**. This claims that patient-centred care is more economically efficient because an approach that encourages individual agency (people doing more for themselves to stay well) is less reliant on expensive interventions. A notable expression of the economic case was the Wanless Review (Wanless, 2002), which deployed economic modelling to argue that the rate of increase in required resources for the NHS would be lower in the "fully engaged scenario" in which people took active responsibility for their own health.
- **The organisational case**. This can be summarised as "happy staff deliver good care", and there is evidence of a positive association – for example in Care Quality Commission reports – between staff satisfaction and patient experience in NHS organisations. In fact, the relationship is unlikely to be just one way. It is likely that there are common factors that nurture both good working conditions and excellent care. The organisational case also draws on the lessons from successive investigations into failures of care, such as in the Mid Staffordshire NHS Foundation Trust; Winterbourne View Hospital, Morecambe Bay Hospital, Gosport Memorial Hospital and Shrewsbury and Telford Hospital NHS Trust. These investigations revealed some common features of organisations

that had delivered poor care, such as autocratic leadership, a lack of focus on quality of care, dysfunctional staff relationships and a failure to listen to the concerns of patients, families and frontline staff.

SECTION 3   A BRIEF HISTORY OF PATIENT-CENTRED CARE

Because the creation of the NHS in 1948 was such an important advance in social welfare, it took decades for a progressive critique of it to gather force. Universal healthcare, available according to need, not means, was – and is – a massive good. But it was not perfect. As Britain moved away from post-war austerity and Edwardian social attitudes, and as healthcare provision expanded and became more technocratic, people began to chafe at medical paternalism, the dominance of "producer" interests and bureaucratic indifference to people's rights.

The 1960s and 1970s. An early turning point was the movement to close down the old asylums and re-provide care for people with mental illness and learning disabilities in the community. As part of broader reorganisations of public services, the 1970s saw the creation of Community Health Councils, which provided a statutory consumer voice in the organisation and delivery of local NHS services.

The 1980s and 1990s. The decades of the Thatcher and Major governments saw a growth in consumerism and a concomitant growing interest in patients having voice, choice and redress when things went wrong. The Griffiths Report (Department of Health and Social Security, 1983), which advised the government on the introduction of modern management into the NHS, argued that the NHS had to recognise and respond to the needs of its "customers". The White Paper "Working for Patients" (Department of Health, 1989) set out the government's intention to introduce market mechanisms into the NHS and cast recipients of healthcare as consumers in an economic sense. The Patient's Charter (Department of Health, 1991), and associated initiatives such as the publication of hospital league tables, further entrenched the view of patients as consumers.

The 2000s. The Blair and Brown governments, initially focussed on increasing investment in the NHS after years of spending restraint, further entrenched patient-centred care in policy, law, guidance and practice. The NHS Plan (Department of Health, 2000) noted that the

NHS ran on an increasingly outdated 1940s model which, among other things, left patients disempowered. It set out a raft of measures, including new patient surveys and hospital-based patient advocates, under which patients would "have a real say in the NHS".

Patient and public engagement or involvement became recognised NHS functions, reflected in job titles. There was growing acknowledgement of the fact that people were living longer and that increasing numbers had to manage long-term conditions, which required a different approach to traditional "patch and mend" medicine. Interest correspondingly grew in models of care for long-term conditions, such as the Wagner Chronic Care Model (Wagner, 2001). The Department of Health launched the Expert Patient Programme (Tidy, 2015). Patient experience was recognised as a key dimension of care quality and started to be systematically surveyed. Meanwhile, many health charities, representing the interests of people with different diseases and conditions, grew in prominence and impact during this time.

The New Labour governments also continued the Conservatives' attachment to market mechanisms and to a view of patients as consumers – reflected, for example, in policies to enable patients to have a choice of hospital. The accumulated advances in patient-centred care were captured in and symbolised by the NHS Constitution, launched in 2009 and updated in 2012, 2015 and 2021 (Department of Health and Social Care, 2021).

The 2010s to present day. The Conservative-led governments from 2010 presided over a much more constrained budget for the NHS. They continued to build patient-centred approaches into law, policy and guidance. The health secretary Andrew Lansley announced his 2010 reform plans with the mantra "no decision about me without me". (This was a borrowing from the disability rights movement and it is debatable whether the policies lived up to this billing.) The Francis Reports into the failures of care in Mid Staffordshire highlighted the importance of NHS organisations listening to patients. The 2014 NHS *Five Year Forward View* (NHS, 2014) heralded the intention of having "a new relationship with patients and communities". The NHS increasingly borrowed empowerment approaches from the more person-centred social care world – for example by encouraging the spread of personal health budgets. And social media provided a fresh fillip to patient-centred activists. But actual empowerment proved more elusive, and in these years the gross inequalities in health highlighted in the seminal 2010 Marmot Review, updated ten years later, continue to provide a grim background to the ever-changing NHS policy scene (Marmot, 2010; Marmot et al., 2020).

A brief review of patient-centred care in other developed countries

Parallel moves towards patient-centred care have occurred in other developed countries. Each country has taken a different path, shaped by the characteristics of how their separate healthcare systems are organised and funded. In Europe the principle of universal coverage holds, which is that all citizens can access healthcare without suffering financial hardship. This is achieved either by giving a strong role to independent health insurance organisations, as in Germany, France and the Netherlands – the "Bismarck" approach – or with governments taking a more central role in both funding and organising healthcare, as in the UK, Italy and Sweden – the "Beveridge" approach.

There is some evidence that Bismarck countries are more patient-centred than Beveridge countries (Health Consumer Powerhouse, 2019). For example, the UK scores well on patient rights and information but poorly on accessibility (waiting times for treatment) and "amber" on outcomes. The Netherlands, on the other hand, score even better on patient rights and information than the UK, and also well on accessibility and outcomes (Health Consumer Powerhouse, 2019).

The Picker Institute notes how Bismarck countries have embedded patient rights in statute. Germany issued a Charter of Rights for People in Need of Long-Term Care and Assistance in 2003. Its Patients' Rights Act of 2013 gives patients explicit rights to choose physicians, hospitals and treatment types, request a second opinion and obtain timely face-to-face information about a proposed treatment. The Dutch have entrenched seven patient rights, similar to those in Germany, with the additional right to coordination between healthcare providers (Paparella, 2016). The NHS in England does have its Constitution, referred to earlier, although the commitments to patients' rights are more modest and less explicit, and balanced by a section on patients' responsibilities.

Uniquely among high-income countries, until recently (with the advent of Obamacare and the Affordable Care Act), there was no attempt at universal coverage in the US. Coverage continues to be offered either through private employment insurance schemes with high levels of co-payments, or through a public safety net for the very poorest and for older people, which leaves millions with inadequate or no cover. Not surprisingly, and despite spending far more overall on healthcare than all other comparable countries, the US scores badly on measures of patient-centred care. In a study comparing eleven high-income countries carried out by the Commonwealth Fund (Schneider et al., 2017) the US comes last on access and equity. Its system has been described as "islands of excellence in a sea of misery" (Pollock, 2011).

Despite the sea of misery, the islands of US excellence do offer examples to other countries and opportunities for them to learn. Being often at the cutting edge of high-tech healthcare, the US has fostered a lively discourse about the downsides of modern medicine and what to do about them. For example, Michael Betz and Lenahan O'Connell (2003) write about the growth of professionalisation, specialisation, bureaucracy and population mobility, and how these have intruded into doctor/patient relationships and left patients feeling powerless and disaffected. Richard Bohmer (2009) argues that patient care has become the domain and responsibility not just of the individual practitioner, but of the whole organisation.

The US has also been at the forefront of practical moves to develop integrated and patient-centred care (for example, within health maintenance organisations such as the Veterans' Administration and Kaiser Permanente); to advance shared decision-making (for instance, through provisions in the Affordable Care Act) and to integrate patients into quality-improvement initiatives (such as through the work of the internationally respected Institute for Health Improvement).

The American discourse has tended to emphasise the importance of patients having greater choice, control and agency, along the lines of Sherry Arnstein's classic ladder of citizen participation in planning processes (Arnstein, 1969), which we cover in more detail later in this chapter (see Section 4, pp. 15–16). These are important dimensions of patient-centred care but, as this book shows, far from being the only ones.

SECTION 4   HOW PATIENT-CENTRED IS CARE NOW?

Is the NHS more patient-centred now than in 1948? In some respects, almost certainly yes, but the question is not straightforward to answer. There is no single measure of the quality of healthcare. It is measured and assessed in a variety of ways, all of which have methodological strengths and weaknesses, but which, looked at together, paint a picture. Overall, there is evidence that the quality and outcomes of healthcare have improved over recent years, both in the UK and other high-income countries. For example, the Euro Health Consumer Index 2018 reported improvements across Western Europe in the previous twelve-year period, including in the UK, against a basket of measures (Health Consumer Powerhouse, 2018). COVID-19 might subsequently be shown to have slowed or reversed that trend.

When it comes to patient-centred care, the picture is more nuanced. As discussed earlier, patient-centred care is not a single, easily defined thing, but a basket of approaches. Assessing it depends to a great extent on the measures chosen and on how we uncover and interpret people's subjective experiences.

Advances in policy

Certainly, there have been significant advances in legislation, policy, service organisation and professional attitudes, alongside broader societal changes. For example:

- **The case for engaging patients** in decisions about, and the management of their own care is now well established. In part this is because advances in public health and medicine have resulted in many more people living longer but with chronic conditions. Patient engagement is particularly relevant to people living with long-term conditions. The NHS's "comprehensive model of personalised care", which brings together a menu of approaches such as shared decision-making, personalised care planning, supported self-management, social prescribing and personal health budgets, is an example of how patient-centred care is moving into the mainstream (NHS, 2019).
- **The patient point of view** is now recognised as a legitimate and important source of data for monitoring and improving services. Patient and carer experiences are seen as indicators of the extent and quality of patient-centred care. Patient views and experiences are routinely collected in the form of national surveys and local feedback mechanisms. Digital platforms have extended the reach of feedback. For example, the website Care Opinion allows patients and carers to post stories about their experiences and elicit responses from providers. Care Opinion has been adopted as a universal engagement platform by the NHS in Scotland.
- **The active involvement of patients** in the design and delivery of services is now seen as a valuable and legitimate endeavour. This is reflected in the various discourses and models of co-design and co-production – for example, the experience-based co-design toolkit offered by the Point of Care Foundation (n.d.).
- **Social mobilising** has been an emerging strand, with social media providing new platforms on which patient activists can organise. Perhaps the best-known example is offered by the

doctor-turned-terminally-ill cancer patient Kate Granger, who in 2013 was dismayed to encounter healthcare staff who failed to introduce themselves to her when she was being treated in hospital. She launched the #HelloMyNameIs campaign to encourage staff always to introduce themselves.

- **A wider role for citizens in health matters** is built into NHS legislation – for example, the duty of commissioners to consult the public on major service changes – and into governance – for example, the role of governors and members of Foundation Trusts, and lay members of clinical commissioning groups. The local public watchdog role once performed by Community Health Councils is now exercised by a network of local Healthwatch organisations.

- **There was a marked "Mid Staffs" effect** as a result of the two inquiries by Robert Francis into poor care at Mid Staffordshire NHS Foundation Trust between 2005 and 2009. The first report (Mid Staffordshire NHS Foundation Trust Public Inquiry, 2010) highlighted multiple failures in a Stafford hospital to attend to the safety and quality of care for patients, and to listen to patients and their families. The second report (Mid Staffordshire NHS Foundation Trust Public Inquiry, 2013) exposed wider systemic failures which enabled that scandal and which made the NHS vulnerable to other similar situations in the future.

    The inquiries prompted soul-searching in the health community about patient focus, patient safety, organisational culture and the importance of accountable and compassionate leadership. The second inquiry gave rise to a significant policy response from the coalition government, with an initial document called "Putting Patients First". Subsequent measures included: a renewal of the inspection and regulation regime under a revamped Care Quality Commission (CQC), the creation of the NHS Leadership Academy, a new duty of candour (in the event of harm suffered by patients or near misses) and a fresh emphasis on listening to patients – symbolised by the introduction of the NHS feedback tool, the "Friends and Family Test". Naomi Chambers and colleagues (Chambers et al., 2018) found that in response to Francis there had been mostly positive (though variable) improvements in the behaviour of boards of NHS organisations.

Advances in practice

How far have these developments in thinking and policy been reflected in healthcare practice and in people's experiences of care? The stories we share in this book present a mix of both good and bad experiences of care. Official data and assessments paint a similar, varied picture. The annual State of Care report published by the health and care regulator the Care Quality Commission is a case in point. In its report for 2019/2020 (CQC, 2020a) the Care Quality Commission assesses most of the care it sees in England as of good quality but also highlights a number of continuing concerns that predate the COVID-19 pandemic:

- The poorer quality of care that is harder to plan for
- The need for care to be delivered in a more joined-up way
- The continued fragility of adult social care provision
- The struggles of the poorest services to make any improvement
- Significant gaps in access to good-quality care, especially mental healthcare
- Persistent inequalities in some aspects of care

In addition the Care Quality Commission notes that while overall quality has been maintained, there was no overall improvement compared with the previous year. It also points out that the pandemic has put further strain on the system and magnified pre-existing inequalities. There is a good deal of continuity between one Care Quality Commission annual report and the next. In its previous report, for 2018/2019, the Care Quality Commission drew attention to problems including widespread difficulties in getting appointments and access to care; a lack of suitable, community-based services, especially for people with a learning disability, autism or mental illness; and people having to fight and "chase" to get the care they need. These can, among other things, be fairly read as deficiencies in patient-centredness. They partly reflect financial pressures and workforce shortages faced by the NHS, but culture, leadership and management also play a part.

The website Quality Watch keeps track of more than 200 indicators of quality of care, including patient experience measures that are relevant to patient-centred care. A similar mixed picture of good and bad emerges in relation to whether patients are informed about medication side effects, feel involved in decisions about their care, feel supported to manage their long-term condition, or report an overall good experience. The typical picture is that the majority report good experiences, but a significant minority do not; the patterns have remained broadly stable over several years but have shown a deterioration more recently. For example, the 2018 adult inpatient survey reported decreased patient experience scores compared with the previous year, in nineteen of the twenty questions asked (NHS, 2019). The 2019 adult inpatient survey

(CQC, 2020b) showed a mixture of improvement and decline against key measures of patient experience.

The charity coalition National Voices published an overview of the state of person-centred care in 2017, drawing on a range of data sources and focussing on a small number of key ingredients of person-centred care: how people experienced information, communication, participation in decisions, care planning and care coordination. It also looked at families and carers. Again, the results were mixed and the report notes that for some aspects of person-centredness – for example, coordination of care – there were no adequate measures (National Voices, 2017).

National Voices also looked at the variations in experience. People's experiences vary depending on time, place and many other factors, but survey data also show some broader patterns in the variability of experience based on demographic group and health status. For example, in the 2018 adult inpatient survey (NHS England, 2019), people with a long-standing health condition had significantly lower experience scores than those with no long-standing condition, and people from certain ethnic groups: for example, Indian, Pakistani, White and Black Caribbean, had significantly lower scores than the White British group (conversely, White Irish and African patients overall had more positive experiences). A 2016 thematic review by the Care Quality Commission (CQC, 2016) highlighted concerns that certain groups were less likely to be sufficiently involved in choices and decisions about their care and treatment – including people with long-term conditions, people over 75, people with dementia, young people with complex health needs, people with a learning disability and people detained under the Mental Health Act or experiencing a mental health crisis.

While it is important to attend to the groups who report worse experiences, there is also learning from what works well. For example, a 2017 report by the Care Quality Commission provides case studies of services that they rated "outstanding" and notes some common characteristics:

> Good leadership is a central part of improvement – services that improve tend to have leaders who are visible and accountable to staff, promote an open and positive organisational culture, and engage effectively with partners. Improvements in the quality of care people are receiving are happening despite tight financial constraints and increased demand across the sectors. Also important is the way that care services in an area work together. (CQC, 2017: 5)

Why isn't the NHS more patient-centred?

After many years of policy designed to make healthcare more patient-centred, the evidence would bear the conclusion that practice lags behind the good intentions. Why is this? A principal reason is that patient-centred care is hard to do, especially hard to do well, and that there are obstacles in the way.

One obstacle is that of capacity. Patient-centred care requires people, money, kit and expertise. A fully patient-centred NHS would, for example, have enough people and resources to devote sufficient time to patients; would train healthcare professionals in shared decision-making and health coaching; have IT systems that allowed patient records to be shared between different hospitals; have simple, effective and welcoming complaints and feedback systems; have the organisational nous to be able to coordinate services seamlessly across a large geography, and so forth. In reality, people, money and kit are always in short supply. So is the expertise needed to run the large and highly complex system which is the NHS. Translating high-level policy into practice challenges even the ablest. And highly able managers and leaders are a strictly finite resource.

Another obstacle is power. Patient-centred care demands a bigger say for patients. In this respect it challenges the current distribution of power and that challenge is to an extent resisted. Power lies predominantly with the government, the managerial senior leadership of the NHS and the health professional elites. The policies and activities of the NHS reflect the priorities of the powerful. These priorities certainly reflect and overlap with the priorities of patients and the public. But they are not the same. In this analysis, the powerful have a strong incentive to maintain their power and are reluctant to share it, so that processes and mechanisms designed to share power are prevented from realising their full radical potential.

The result is that patients – and also frontline staff – can often feel powerless. They can experience engagement efforts as tokenistic or paternalistic: the doctor who is not really listening, the public consultation designed to rubber-stamp decisions already made behind closed doors. In terms of an analysis of power (and how far it is shared with the citizenry), the charge is that the NHS remains stuck at best on the middle ("tokenism") rungs of Arnstein's famous ladder of participation (Arnstein, 1969).

While those with power can choose to share it, they can also wrest it back. In that sense, without more radical change, patient-centredness remains provisional. During the COVID-19 pandemic, a number of

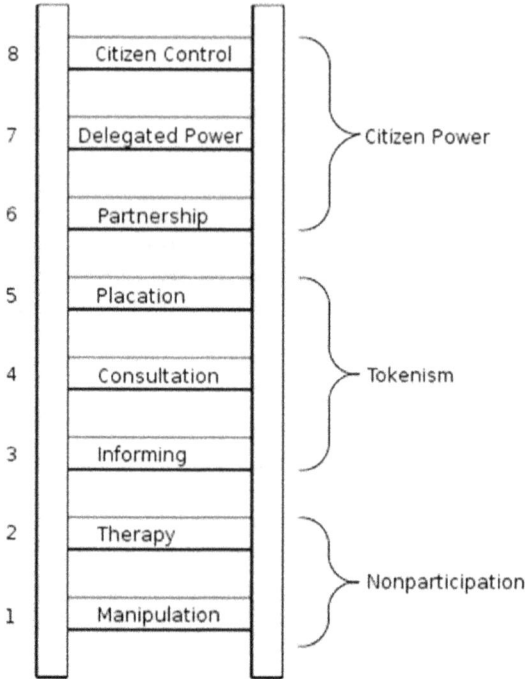

Figure 1.1   Arnstein's ladder of participation

patient organisations noted that major changes were made to the way in which the NHS was organised, with little or no involvement of communities and public representatives. When the going gets tough, patient and public engagement can be seen as a "nice to have", rather than an essential ingredient of informed decision-making.

This power imbalance cannot be fully understood unless also viewed through the lens of equality, diversity and inclusion. In important respects those at the top of the NHS do not represent the communities they serve, and from which the broader NHS workforce is drawn. Ethnicity is the most visible (though far from the only) point of difference. The report on the "snowy white peaks" of the NHS (Kline, 2014) highlighted the persistent lack of ethnic diversity in the upper echelons of NHS management and explored the connections between this lack of diversity; the experiences of inequality and discrimination among Black, Asian and minority ethnic staff; and shortcomings in patient care. Race inequality was further highlighted in 2020 as a result of the unequal impacts of the COVID-19 pandemic, and because of the worldwide Black Lives Matters protests following the murder of George Floyd in the US. There is growing debate about such concepts as unconscious bias, white privilege and intersectionality, and their applicability in the healthcare context. In the longer run, for example through the application of the NHS Workforce Race Equality Standard, it is to be hoped that an NHS leadership which better reflects the communities it serves might also better hear those communities.

A further obstacle is that of NHS organisational culture. Commentators and academics such as Professor Michael West have highlighted enduring features of NHS culture that are likely to stand in the way of achieving patient-centred care (West, 2017). A top-down, authoritarian style of management is seen as widespread: one that focusses more on managing performance and hitting targets than on engagement and improvement, and which can stifle innovation and the adoption and spread of good practice. The aforementioned Francis Inquiries into the poor care at Mid Staffordshire NHS Foundation Trust (Mid Staffordshire NHS Foundation Trust Public Inquiry, 2010 and 2013) shone a light on the impact of this management style, sparking a wider discourse about NHS culture at its most dysfunctional, where forceful management veers into bullying, intimidation and victimisation, a failure to listen to patients and frontline staff, and with failures of care denied and covered up.

It goes without saying that such authoritarian cultures are conducive neither to patient-centred care nor to staff empowerment. Disempowered and disaffected staff are not in the best position to provide good care. Nor are they well placed to act as respected and supported champions for change and improvement. In an adverse culture which is potentially or actually harmful to patients, staff have limited options. They can speak up, but that is risky for them. The whistleblowing option is frequently a career-ending one. They can keep their heads down and do their jobs as best they can. They can give up trying to make things better, even within their direct sphere of influence, and adopt a stance of "learned helplessness". Or they can quit.

A key response to problems of NHS culture has been to seek improvements in the quality of NHS leadership. This was a significant motivation for the creation of the NHS Leadership Academy in 2013, with its emphasis on nurturing a new cadre of open, engaging, collaborative and compassionate NHS leaders.

The annual NHS staff survey provides some evidence that NHS culture and leadership are improving. The results of the 2019 survey show a slowly improving trend on many of the measures, but with some areas of continuing concern. Thus there has been a significant rise in the proportion of staff who would recommend their organisation as a place to work, but more than a third (37 per cent) still would not. There has been a small rise in the proportion of staff who say that they would feel secure reporting concerns about unsafe clinical practice, but 28 per cent say they would not (NHS England, 2020).

Open and compassionate local NHS leaders may find themselves in conflict with national NHS bosses. The dictates of quality may, for example, be in tension with the dictates of financial management. To this extent, the perspectives of culture and power intermingle. The top-down, target-driven NHS management culture is very much an outcome of priorities set by government ministers, and how hard these priorities are driven. The imposition of power from Whitehall can foster power-lessness on the wards and in the clinics.

Conversely, the perspectives of capacity, power and culture offer hope. The NHS is shaped by powerful political and economic forces but it is also the cumulative effort of millions of staff. To differing extents, everyone in the NHS has the scope to improve their capacity to be patient-centred, to confront or share power and to improve the culture of their teams and organisations. The stories in this book illus-trate some of the possibilities.

SECTION 5   STORYTELLING: THE APPROACH WE TAKE IN THIS BOOK

There is no way to understand the human world without stories. Stories are everywhere. Stories are us. (Storr, 2019: 2)

This book is based on stories. Storytelling draws on lay wisdom to gener-ate new understandings. It complements and enriches the knowledge that comes from science and data. Storytelling is as old as humanity. In the forms of myths, legends and fables it was the means by which groups and societies transmitted their histories, identities, moralities and cul-tural meanings. The words "story" and "history" are closely related and, in some languages (for example French and German), identical (*histoire, Geschichte*).

While in contemporary culture we often associate story with enter-tainment, it has always served a serious purpose too. Stories have power. They create an immersive experience for listeners and readers which can be more compelling and memorable than factual information (Mar and Oatley, 2008). Artur Lugmayr and colleagues (2016: 15709 and

15715) discuss the concept of "serious storytelling" in which the power of narrative – conveying experience, triggering emotional responses and reshaping understandings – is used to achieve serious goals. Organisations are formed and reformed in part by the stories which members tell about their collective selves, values, victories and challenges (Seely-Brown et al., 2005).

Stories can be a call to action, part of social mobilising for change. Marshall Ganz, who heavily influenced Barack Obama, and has also worked with the NHS, wrote:

> A story is like a poem. It moves not by how long it is, nor how eloquent or complicated. It moves by offering an experience or moment through which we grasp the feeling or insight the poet communicates. The more specific the details we choose to recount, the more we can move our listeners, the more powerfully we can articulate our values. (Ganz, 2008)

Storytelling in healthcare and in the NHS

The Victorian physician Sir William Osler, an early enthusiast for hearing the patient story, stressed the centrality of history-taking: "Just listen to your patient, he is telling you the diagnosis." He helped influence the course of undergraduate and postgraduate medical education (Bliss, 1999). Michael Balint talks about the "flash of understanding" that arises in medical consultations as a result of close listening and probing questioning of the patient (Balint, 1967). Stories are increasingly a feature in modern healthcare. This reflects the rise of service user and survivor movements and a growing interest in patient-centred care. It could also reflect an impulse to restore the human into what some see as an emotionally distant and over-technocratic culture in modern healthcare. Patient stories are appear more often in healthcare literature, such as the growing "single testimony" literature by frontline clinicians – for example, Henry Marsh (2014), Adam Kay (2017), Christie Watson (2018) and Rachel Clarke (2020) – and in books on dying by Atul Gawande (2015) and Kathryn Mannix (2017), and on mental ill health by Linda Gask (2015) and Suzanne O'Sullivan (2015).

Storytelling can be a teaching instrument (Rossiter, 2002). Organisations like Healthtalk (www.healthtalk.org) and Patient Voices (www. patientvoices.org.uk) use stories to help patients understand their conditions and to support organisations to change their cultures and behaviours in light of people's experiences. Enza Gucciardi and colleagues

(2016) discuss how stories can be used to encourage behaviour change and support people to manage their long-term health conditions. Mark Exworthy (2011) examines how health service managers can come to change their professional understandings and practices as a result of recounting and reflecting on their own personal experiences of illness and healthcare. It is now considered good practice to start board meetings of NHS organisations with a patient or staff story in order to keep discussion grounded in what matters at the frontline and to focus minds on care quality. Making use of new media platforms, TEDxNHS (www.tedxnhs.com) was founded in 2016 as a volunteer movement to allow the voices of everyday NHS staff and patients to be heard on a national stage. It aims to break down the walls that can exist between professions, organisations and cultures and to share learning in a new and engaging way.

In short, storytelling has secured a well-recognised place in health and sickness discourses – a status analogous to that of oral history in relation to academic history. In parallel, and in the form of "narrative research", storytelling has established legitimacy as a social science research method, as argued by Trish Greenhalgh and Tom Wengraf (2008), for instance. There is a standing critique of the narrative method as "anecdotal" and thus insufficiently scientific (Exworthy, 2011), but this is changing. For example, Rachel Rose and colleagues (2015), synthesising a large body of evidence, showed that patient stories had the potential to facilitate culture change, more patient-centred practices and greater humanism in healthcare.

Finding stories: Problems of ethics and methodology

In Chapters 2 to 7 of this book we present stories that we have collected, curated and then presented in ways that are intended to promote reflection and learning. The Appendix at the very end of the book has the complete anonymised list of interviewees, including background details. This method is distinct from the "single testimony" accounts we have described above. The storytellers did not approach and use us as a vehicle for disseminating their story. Rather, we initiated and controlled the process. As authors we are intermediaries between the people with stories and the people who might learn from these stories. This process raises a number of considerations which are both ethical and methodological.

There is first the question of selection bias. For example, in finding people to tell their stories it is relatively easy to draw upon a pool of actively engaged people with strong links into professional circles and thus to exclude voices from poorer, disadvantaged, more diverse and marginalised communities. Further bias is possible in how the authors translate people's experiences into text on a page. Some people have a clear story that they want to tell, but for others it is more a case of responding to an invitation to share their experience, which is then turned into a story through the processes of interview, transcription and editing.

Stories are inherently biased to the extent that they embody the storytellers' values, the limitations of their memories, and their judgements about what is important and what it means. Storytellers select some things, present them in particular ways and exclude other things. There is a risk that authors of a book like this introduce further bias through their active involvement in creating and presenting the stories. At best we are neutral brokers between storyteller and audience, but we risk distorting or misrepresenting our volunteers and at worst exploiting them.

A third issue is the risk that storytellers suffer in the process of telling their story. Though recounting a difficult or traumatic experience can be therapeutic, the opposite can also be true. Inviting people to reveal their private thoughts and feelings, as distinct from a more "public account" can be challenging (Cornwell, 1984). Putting a traumatic experience into words is not always possible or helpful (Van der Kolk, 2014; Hooper, 2019). Patients sometimes express frustration that they have told their story repeatedly but nothing has changed as a result (whether in the context of research or in service improvement). It can be argued that hearing a patient story confers a moral obligation to act in light of it.

These ethical risks informed our methodological approach, including our consent process. To minimise selection bias and maximise diversity, we reached out in a variety of different ways and sought individuals of varying ages, backgrounds and health issues. We found it relatively straightforward to achieve a spread of ages, a gender balance and a degree of ethnic diversity. It took more effort to compensate for the bias towards people from middle-class, professional circles (for example, those who are well connected with the health world, and those with whom the authors had a personal connection). It was hardest of all to find people who were not already in some way engaged, either as health volunteers (such as chairing a GP patient participation group) or more broadly active in their communities. As a reminder, a table summarising our storytellers and some of their characteristics, appropriately anonymised, is shown in the Appendix.

We used a variant of Wengraf's (2001) biographic narrative method – essentially asking people to tell their story in the way they wanted to, which was often "from the beginning", wherever that was, with only minimal prompts from us along the way. Our stories were gathered through a mixture of face-to-face and telephone interviews. The interviews were recorded. As listeners, we were sensitive to the possibility that storytellers become emotionally distressed in their recounting and were always ready to pause or end the interview. (This did not happen.)

The listening process was constantly interesting for us as interviewers. There were various aspects that on reflection we thought were of wider relevance to the art of listening to patients in the NHS:

- Our storytellers spoke freely. They had as much time as they needed (on average about an hour), and as listeners we had no agenda, other than to attend to their account and occasionally nudge it along through our questions and reactions. These are very different conditions from those which characterise typical clinical and other NHS encounters, in which professional listening is for a defined purpose (e.g. diagnosis), is geared towards determining action (e.g. referral) and is under time pressure. We realised that it was a privilege to be able to listen free of the responsibility to do something immediately. It enabled us to give our full attention.

- We were surprised that it was relatively easy to elicit personal accounts over the phone, despite the absence of eye contact and body language.

- Not having to take notes was a further liberation for the listener. It was also experienced by at least one interviewee as more respectful: the professional who is constantly clacking away at a computer or head down in a notebook can often be a source of irritation in a therapeutic context.

- Some tales were fragmented, raw, unvarnished or impressionistic; others were polished narratives. This variation partly reflected the extent to which people had told their story previously. It is also the case that some people are naturally gifted storytellers and others much less so. We realised that all the stories contained important learning, regardless of the communication skills of the interviewee. It reminded us that in the clamour of voices, there lies the risk of paying undue attention to the eloquent and persuasive, to the detriment of the halting and inarticulate.

SECTION 6   HOW TO READ THIS BOOK

There are twenty-five stories in this book, of varying length, divided across six chapters. The chapters group the stories around the major stages of the life-course, from birth to death, and around some of the key categories of ill health. A concluding chapter draws together some of the key issues raised by the stories. Each story chapter begins with a brief introduction to the connecting theme, presents the stories, and then concludes with a short set of questions designed to encourage reflection on the implications of the stories for practice. The stories do not lend themselves to a conventional textbook format in which a body of knowledge is progressively laid out and then translated into key facts, tips and actions. The principal demands that the stories make of the reader are: engage and reflect. It follows that the reader is free to read as few or as many of the chapters as desired, and in any order.

Chapter 2 is about pregnancy and childbirth. **Cathy** is a healthcare professional who recently gave birth. **James** is an older new father.

Chapter 3 is about children and young people. **Dan** is a normally healthy teenager who became acutely ill. His father Jonathan tells the story. **Jim** was a severely disabled young man from birth until his death aged 36. His parents Lucinda and Justin tell his story. **Eve** remembers how as a child she came to be diagnosed with Type 1 diabetes. **Finbar** is a teenage boy with a diagnosis of scoliosis. His mother Eileen tells the story of being his carer.

Chapter 4 is about managing long-term health conditions. **Katie** has had Type 1 diabetes for about twenty-five years. **Tim** is a young man living with epilepsy. **Joanna** has various long-term conditions, including a rare condition. **Jasmin** waited four years to get a diagnosis of lupus. **Venetia** lives with chronic fatigue syndrome.

Chapter 5 is about adult acute care and cancer. **Jill** suffered a major knee injury. **Andrea** had an operation to remove her gallbladder. **Lucy** was hospitalised with sepsis. **Shona** experienced breast cancer.

Chapter 6 is about mental illness. **Audrey** describes her quest to find services for a family member. **Stanley** describes his breakdown and subsequent years of contact with mental health services. **Alan** has been living with bipolar disorder for over twenty years. **Nathan** is a teenager with various mental health issues. **Lucy** is a retired hospital psychiatrist with a severe and enduring mental illness.

Chapter 7 is about older age and end of life. **Robert** is in his 80s with a heart condition and stomach and joint problems. **Rabiya** cares for her mother who has dementia. **James** looked after his mother who had dementia. **Sheila** cares for her husband who has dementia. **Kauri's** dad died of pancreatic cancer.

REFERENCES

Arnstein, S. (1969) "A ladder of citizen participation", *Journal of the American Planning Association* 35 (4): 216–224.

Balint, M. (1957) *The Doctor, his Patient and the Illness* (Pitman: London).

Betz, M. and L. O'Connell (2003) "Changing Doctor–Patient Relationships and the Rise in Concern for Accountability", in P. Conrad and V. Leiter (eds), *Health and Health Care as Social Problems* (Lanham, MD: Rowman & Littlefield).

Bliss, M. (1999) *William Osler: A life in medicine* (Oxford: Oxford University Press).

Bohmer, R. (2009) *Designing Care* (Boston, MA: Harvard Business Press).

Chambers, N., R. Thorlby, A. Boyd, J. Smith, N. Proudlove, H. Kendrick and R. Mannion (2018) *Responses to Francis: Changes in board leadership and governance in acute hospitals in England since 2013*, www.research.manchester.ac.uk/portal/files/66318094/responses_to_francis_report.pdf (accessed 3 January 2021).

Clarke, R. (2020) *Dear Life* (London: Little, Brown).

Cornwell, J. (1984) *Hard-Earned Lives: Accounts of health and illness from East London* (London: Tavistock Publications).

CQC (2017) *Celebrating Good Care, Championing Outstanding Care*, www.cqc.org.uk/sites/default/files/20170420_celebratinggoodcare2017.pdf (accessed 3 January 2021).

CQC (2016) *Better Care in My Hands*, www.cqc.org.uk/sites/default/files/20160519_Better_care_in_my_hands_FINAL.pdf (accessed 3 January 2021).

CQC (2020a) *The State of Health Care and Adult Social Care in England 2019/20*, HC 799 (Newcastle: CQC), www.cqc.org.uk/sites/default/files/20201016_stateofcare1920_fullreport.pdf (accessed 3 January 2021).

CQC (2020b) *Adult Inpatient Survey 2019*, www.cqc.org.uk/sites/default/files/20200702_ip19_statisticalrelease.pdf (accessed 3 January 2021).

Department of Health (1989) "Working for Patients", White Paper, Cm 555 (London: HMSO).

Department of Health (1991) *The Patient's Charter* (London: HMSO).

Department of Health (2000) *The NHS Plan: A plan for investment, a plan for reform*, Cm 4818-I 2000 (London: Stationery Office).

Department of Health (2011) *NHS Patient Experience Framework*, https://assets.publishing.service.gov.uk/government/uploads/system/uploads/attachment_data/file/215159/dh_132788.pdf (accessed 3 January 2021).

Department of Health and Social Security (1983) *NHS Management Inquiry* (Griffiths Report) (London: HMSO).

Department of Health and Social Care (2021) *The NHS Constitution in England* https://www.gov.uk/government/publications/the-nhs-constitution-for-england (accessed 21 March 2021).

Exworthy, M. (2011) "The illness narrative of health managers: developing an analytical framework", *Evidence & Policy* 7 (3): 345–358.

Ganz, M. (2008) "What Is Public Narrative?" working paper, https://changemakerspodcast.org/wp-content/uploads/2017/09/Ganz-WhatIsPublicNarrative08.pdf (accessed 3 January 2021).

Gask, L. (2015) *The Other Side of Silence* (Chichester: Summersdale).

Gawande, A. (2015) *Being Mortal* (London: Profile Books).

Greenhalgh, T. and T. Wengraf (2008) "Collecting stories: is it research? Is it good research? Preliminary guidance based on a Delphi study", *Medical Education* 42: 242–247.

Gucciardi, E., N. Jean-Pierre, G. Karam et al. (2016) "Designing and delivering facilitated storytelling interventions for chronic disease self-management: a scoping review", *BMC Health Services Research* 16 (249), https://bmchealthservices.biomedcentral.com/articles/10.1186/s12913-016-1474-7 (accessed 3 January 2021).

Health Consumer Powerhouse (2019) *Euro Health Consumer Index 2018*, https://healthpowerhouse.com/media/EHCI-2018/EHCI-2018-report.pdf (accessed 3 January 2021).

Health Foundation (2016) *Person Centred Care Made Simple*, www.health.org.uk/sites/default/files/PersonCentredCareMadeSimple_0.pdf (accessed 3 January 2021).

Hooper, C. A. (2019) *On Routine Enquiry: Reflections from the evaluation of the Visible project*, https://visibleproject.org.uk/wp-content/uploads/2020/02/On-Routine-Enquiry-Jan2020.pdf (accessed 16 April 2021).

Kay, A. (2017) *This Is Going to Hurt* (London: Picador).

Kline, R. (2014) *The "Snowy White Peaks" of the NHS: A survey of discrimination in governance and leadership and the potential impact on patient care in London and England* (London: Middlesex University), www.mdx.ac.uk/_data/assets/pdf_file/0015/50190/The-snowy-white-peaks-of-the-NHS.pdf (accessed 5 January 2021).

Lugmayr, A., E. Sutinen, J. Suhonen, H. Hlavacs, C.I. Sedano and C.S. Montero (2017) "Serious storytelling – a first definition and review", *Multimedia Tools and Applications* 76: 15707–15733.

Mannix, K. (2017) *With the End in Mind* (London: William Collins)

Mar, R. and K. Oatley (2008) "The function of fiction is the abstraction and simulation of social experience", *Association for Psychological Science* 3(3): 173–192.

Marmot, M. (2010) *Fair Society, Healthy Lives: Strategic review of health inequalities in England, post-2010* (London: Marmot Review).

Marmot, M., J. Allen, T. Boyce, P. Goldblatt and J. Morrison (2020) *Health Equity in England: The Marmot Review 10 years on* (London: Health Foundation), www.health.org.uk/publications/reports/the-marmot-review-10-years-on (accessed 5 January 2021).

Marsh, H. (2014) *Do No Harm* (London: Weidenfeld and Nicolson).

Mid Staffordshire NHS Foundation Trust Public Inquiry (2010) *Independent Inquiry into Care Provided by Mid Staffordshire NHS Foundation Trust, January 2005 to March 2009*, 2 vols (the first Francis Inquiry), HC 375 (London: Stationery Office), www.gov.uk/government/publications/independent-inquiry-into-care-provided-by-mid-staffordshire-nhs-foundation-trust-january-2001-to-march-2009 (accessed 5 January 2021).

Mid Staffordshire NHS Foundation Trust Public Inquiry (2013) *Report of the Mid Staffordshire NHS Foundation Trust Public Inquiry* (the second Francis Inquiry), HC 947 (London: Stationery Office), https://assets.publishing.service.gov.uk/government/uploads/system/uploads/attachment_data/file/279124/0947.pdf (accessed 3 January 2021).

National Voices (2017) *Person-Centred Care in 2017: Evidence from service users*, www.nationalvoices.org.uk/sites/default/files/public/publications/person-centred_care_in_2017_-_national_voices.pdf (accessed 3 January 2021).

NHS (2019) *Comprehensive Model of Personalised Care*, www.england.nhs.uk/publication/comprehensive-model-of-personalised-care/ (accessed 3 January 2021).

NHS England (2014) *Five Year Forward View*, www.england.nhs.uk/wp-content/uploads/2014/10/5yfv-web.pdf (accessed 3 January 2021).

NHS England (2019) *Statistical Bulletin: Overall patient experience scores 2018 adult inpatient survey update*, www.england.nhs.uk/statistics/wp-content/uploads/sites/2/2019/06/Bulletin_2018_IP_FINAL.pdf (accessed 4 January 2021).

NHS England (2020) *NHS Staff Survey 2019: National results briefing*, www.nhsstaffsurveys.com/Caches/Files/ST19_National%20briefing_FINAL%20V2.pdf (accessed 3 January 2021).

O'Sullivan, S. (2015) *It's All in Your Head* (London: Vintage).

Paparella, G. (2016) *Patient-Centred Care in Europe: A cross-country comparison of health system performance, strategies and structures* (Oxford: Picker Institute Europe).

Point of Care Foundation (n.d.): "Evidence and resources: toolkit", www.pointofcarefoundation.org.uk/evidence-resources/ (accessed 3 January 2021).

Pollock, A. (2011) "Competition in health care: the risks", A Better NHS, 29 June, https://abetternhs.net/2011/06/29/competition/ (accessed 3 January 2021).

Rose, R., S. Chakraborty, P. Mason-Lai, W. Brocke, S. Page and D, Cawthorpe (2016) "The storied mind: a meta-narrative review exploring the capacity of stories to foster humanism in health care", *Journal of Hospital Administration* 5 (1): 52–61.

Rossiter, M. (2002) "Narrative and stories in adult teaching and learning: ERIC Digest", *Educational Resources Information Center Digest* ED473147, https://files.eric.ed.gov/fulltext/ED473147.pdf (accessed 3 January 2021).

Schneider, E., D. Sarnak, D. Squires, A. Shah and M. Doly (2017) *Mirror, Mirror: How the US health care system compares internationally at a time of radical change* (New York: Commonwealth Fund).

Seely-Brown, J., S. Denning, K. Groh and L. Prusak (2005) *Storytelling in Organizations: Why storytelling is transforming 21st century organizations and management* (Oxford: Elsevier Butterworth Heinemann).

Storr, W. (2019) *The Science of Storytelling* (London: HarperCollins).

Tidy, C. (2015) "Expert patients", Patient, 8 May, https://patient.info/doctor/expert-patients (accessed 5 January 2021).

Van der Kolk, B. (2014) *The Body Keeps the Score: Mind, brain and body in the transformation of trauma* (London: Penguin).

Wagner, E.H., B.T. Austin, C. Davis, M. Hindmarsh, J. Schaefer and A. Bonomi (2001) "Improving chronic illness care: translating evidence into action", *Health Affairs* 20 (6): 64–78.

Wanless, D. (2002) *Securing Our Future Health: Taking a long-term view* (London: HM Treasury).

Watson, C. (2018) *The Language of Kindness* (London: Chatto and Windus).

Wengraf, T. (2001) *Qualitative Research Interviewing: Biographic narrative and semi-structured methods* (London: Sage).

West, M. (2017) *Caring to Change* (London: King's Fund).

PREGNANCY AND CHILDBIRTH

INTRODUCTION

This chapter contains two stories about pregnancy and childbirth. The first story is told by Cathy, a healthcare professional who became pregnant and then had a difficult time when she gave birth. In the second story we hear from James about becoming a new dad. We come across James again when he tells of his experiences of caring for his mother with dementia in Chapter 7. As we do in other chapters, at the end we pose questions arising from these stories, to simulate your thinking and reflection.

Pregnancy and childbirth are natural processes which nevertheless carry medical risk for mother and baby. Women demand choice and control in maternity services and at the same time expect safe and expert care. The recent history of maternity services in the UK can be read as the interplay between these two factors. From the 1960s there was a growth in activism in opposition to what was seen as the excessive medicalisation of pregnancy and childbirth. The National Childbirth Trust (NCT, www.nct.org.uk), founded in 1956, was central to this movement.

The landmark *Changing Childbirth* report (Department of Health, 1993) paved the way for shifts in policy and practice, including a greater emphasis on the availability of midwife-led care and more choice for women about the place of birth. General practice was also trying to listen more carefully to what women wanted (see, for example, Mellor and Chambers, 1995). In the ensuing decades, there were many improvements in the quality and outcomes of maternity care. For instance, the stillbirth and neonatal mortality rates in England fell by over 20 per cent between 2006 and 2016.

But problems remain and new challenges have emerged. More women have children at an older age. More women have complex health needs that may affect their pregnancy, their well-being and that of their baby. A recent report from researchers at Oxford University found that black women in the UK are five times more likely to die in pregnancy or childbirth, compared with white women. Asian women are twice as likely to die compared to white women (Knight et al., 2019). In the US black and indigenous Americans are two to three times more likely to die from pregnancy-related causes than white women (Petersen et al., 2019).

In addition, there have been scandals of poor and unsafe maternity care, as evidenced by the Morecambe Bay public inquiry (Morecambe Bay Investigation, 2015) and the continuing inquiry into care at Shrewsbury and Telford Hospitals NHS Trust (Ockenden Report, 2020). Hundreds of millions of pounds are spent every year compensating families for negligence during maternity care. Meanwhile, women can still find that they are denied choice and control when it comes to critical decisions about their care. These issues were considered in the *National Maternity Review* (NHS England, 2016), which set out a renewed vision for personalised, woman-centred, kinder and more professional maternity services in England.

THE STORIES

In Chapter 1 (Section 2, p. 4) we offer an understanding of patient-centred care in general as:

- Understanding and valuing what matters to patients
- Seeing the whole person
- Respecting people's rights and autonomy
- Being customer focussed

The policy rhetoric and the reality for women don't yet match up, according to the numerous care failings and the reviews mentioned above. The stories below contain further examples of shortcomings, as well as good practices. They also suggest prompts for policymakers, professionals and NHS managers to take action.

A literally life-changing event, giving birth is seemingly rarely straightforward. The two stories presented below testify to that. **Cathy**'s is a longer story because so much happened to her. **James** narrates the events of the birth of both of his children, but altogether this is a shorter piece. In Chapter 3, the story of **Jim**, Lucinda and Justin (Story 4, pp. 61–73) includes a description of what happened when Lucinda gave birth to Jim, who had severe congenital physical and learning disabilities. All three examples demonstrate what a huge difference it makes to parents if health services are responsive when things don't go according to plan.

Story 1: Cathy

Cathy had complications in pregnancy and labour and needed an emergency caesarean section. Her postnatal care was also full of incident: her wound became infected and she had to be readmitted to hospital. By profession Cathy is a critical care nurse, and this undoubtedly shaped her expectations, her experiences and her subsequent reflections on them. Overall, she believes she received good care, with some lapses. Her story is quite a rollercoaster and the reader might be left taking a view different to Cathy's own.

Cathy: My account relates to the antenatal care and labour care of the birth of my son, who is nearly six months old now. I had a lot of complications and difficulties throughout the birth particularly, but I believe in general I received really excellent care, although I had a really tough time. I think the fact that I'm a healthcare practitioner myself allows me to realise that even though things were going horribly wrong, I was receiving really good care. So basically from the start, all my midwife appointments before I had my son were excellent because I saw the same person every single time. And having talked to a lot of other people about that, they saw a different midwife every single time. I felt like I had a real relationship, a real bond with the midwife, she was really exceptional and made me feel very comfortable. Unfortunately, during my pregnancy I was pregnant with twins and I lost one of the twins.

It's fine, it was right at the start but I was therefore very nervous and very anxious about the process and she was fantastic at reassuring me the whole way through. And I think because I'm a critical care nurse, I work in ICU [Intensive Care Unit], I always see the dangers and the difficulties around everything. I always assume the worst, not the best. So I was very much risk aware. And so, a lot of people want to go to the birth centre and have a lovely birth with the candles and all that kind of thing, but I really really didn't want to do that. And she listened to me and guided me though the steps, if you know what I mean.

So in some ways being a healthcare professional made things harder for you because you were more conscious of the risks and what could go wrong?

C: Absolutely. Because I go to all of the emergencies, I only see things while the emergency bell is pulled and everyone goes running. So I never see the lovely births, I only see the ones that go horribly wrong, and she was really good at listening to me. She was a very senior midwife, in fact she was promoted during our time together, so she should have stopped seeing patients. But I think because we'd had such a bond, she said, I'd like to see you but would you mind coming outside my working hours.

Did you ever get the sense you were getting a special service because you work in the NHS, or would that have happened anyway?

C: It's a good question. I think possibly, but she did say that she kept other patients on, other mothers on as well, that she didn't really want to give them up. So I think that she was a really exceptional midwife but also possibly had difficulties giving up her workload and doing her new role maybe.

One thing I really relished was her talking to me as a fellow health professional, and not talking down to me but also appreciating that I knew very little about midwifery. It was a relationship which I thought was very much built on mutual respect.

So I had fantastic antenatal care. And then when I went into labour things started going wrong. When I started having contractions, I couldn't feel the baby at all, couldn't feel that he was moving, and you are supposed to feel the movements. And so they told me to come into hospital to be checked and actually he was fine but they said, because you have reduced movements you can't go home. So then for several hours things passed very normally and my waters broke. And then I felt incredibly shivery, I just didn't feel right at all, and this is the one of two times I feel that I had poor care.

My midwife who had been looking after me was on her break, so I spoke to one of the other midwives and I said, look, I just don't feel right, can you please check my temperature, I think I'm having rigors [severe shivers and high fever]. And she said, oh no, it's just because your waters have broken, da da da, and refused to do it. I did feel uncomfortable saying, I'm a nurse so you should do this. And I kind of let myself be talked round because, you know, I'd never been in labour before, I'd never done any midwifery. But actually when she came back and I still felt dreadful, I spoke to my other midwife, she did my observations straightaway and it turns out that I had sepsis. So actually there was quite a big window of time in which I could have been treated and I wasn't treated and I felt quite upset about that.

But when I actually got the care for the sepsis, it was excellent. And there is a sepsis pathway which is six steps that you should do within a certain amount of time and they did all of those. Because I know from my experience that quite often it's done quite shoddily, I felt very comfortable with that care particularly, that they were doing it correctly.

How bad a mistake was it not responding to your reports of feeling feverish?

C: Well, it could have been quite bad because the Surviving Sepsis Campaign shows that if you act within the first hour of having a temperature then you've got a much improved outcome for the patient. So she really drove down the clock on that.

So having a temperature is a serious sign in labour?

C: Yes it is, alongside several other things. So I feel that that it could have been an opportunity missed and if I wasn't a nurse myself and pushed the point and it happened to somebody else, they may not have received that care. And my labour had to be sped up because they were so scared about my son receiving the infection. Luckily he didn't, but had that been delayed then maybe he would. I certainly wasn't listened to and I don't think that was acceptable then.

But then, I know that actually people are absolutely stretched. It was a weekend, there was a ward full of people in labour, the other midwife was on her break. I can completely understand, a lady saying I don't feel quite right, and her knowing that my waters have broken, I can understand why that happened. It was just frustrating, I'd say.

I suppose a lot of the judgement of healthcare professionals is making the distinction between I don't feel that great and this is a warning sign.

C: Yes, definitely.

And it must be quite difficult to make that distinction sometimes?

C: Yes, absolutely and I'm sure that quite often women in labour aren't the most rational people who make salient points about their clinical state. So I can completely understand why that happened but I do think that, given that I'd come in with reduced movements of my baby, that

I clearly said I feel like I have a high temperature, it's a two-second job that would have said either way, whether I was right or not, and that should have happened.

Apart from that time, I did feel generally well looked after. They brought me pain relief when I asked, they said that they would come back and do monitoring of the baby: they said, I'll be back in about an hour and generally they were. So it didn't feel understaffed, it felt that they had a really good service. And another point, I think that they were generally quite good at managing expectations. It's one of the really big things in healthcare that people are, like, I'll be back but don't give you a timescale. But actually they were very good at saying, we are going to do this and then that and they stuck to it and if they didn't they came and explained why. And I thought that that was excellent.

Being reliable, doing what you said you were going to do, is probably one of the things that contributes to a sense of being properly looked after.

C: Absolutely. And if you're not going to deliver what you said you would deliver, coming in and explaining before the patient asks is such an important part of it, because otherwise they feel like they are bugging you and they are chasing you … they can't relax because they need to be on your case. If you actually can manage their expectations appropriately, then those people relax. When I felt well looked after in my labour, I relaxed a lot more and it was a lot easier. And so it actually feels like it had, not even just an effect on my emotional well-being, physically my blood pressure would have been better, et cetera.

Yes, it's really interesting this whole business about managing expectations and the link with how anxious or calm you are, and then the link to how well you can respond to care.

C: Yeah, one of my jobs is to look after deteriorating patients on the ward. So I meet a lot of disgruntled patients who say, God, well I have been telling the nurses for hours that I don't feel right. And quite often going down to the root cause, it's because the nurse has said she will do something and hasn't and hasn't managed that expectation appropriately. You can look at the board and see the under-staffing and you can understand why. But if she had just popped her head around the corner and said, I know I need to do that thing, I will be right back with you – that one sentence would have a huge impact on a patient. I don't think that that is understood really in practice.

So after that point they started monitoring me all the time. And there was a couple of times when the baby's heart rate dropped considerably, so they realised that they needed to speed up my labour. They needed to start me on a drip of oxytocin which speeds up your contractions, to try and make you have a quicker natural labour. And for that you should ideally have an epidural. So I was moved up to labour ward; that process took longer than it should have done, but they were completely full and explained to me why that happened and that was absolutely fine. I still received good enough care and they explained to me why that was. But when I eventually went up there, the midwife from the previous ward had said, oh you know you don't want an epidural, it can slow down your labour. But actually I really did want an epidural and I had written that in my birth plan. I am a nurse, I can see how good epidurals are and the labour scared me, the pain of it terrified me.

And because she was so insistent, I kind of said, yeah yeah yeah, not agreeing with her. She then went off and told the ward round that I didn't want an epidural and so when they came in, they said so we've been told by the midwife that you don't want an epidural. I said, that's absolutely not true and that led to quite a big delay in me getting an epidural. So that was the second bit of my care that I think was poor. She had a very clear opinion, which actually doesn't reflect guidelines and policy at all, and she decided that that would be my opinion and then without my consent gave something that was opposite to my wish to the ward round. And I did have a very clear birth plan that said, I would want an epidural in these circumstances.

To what extent did you get a sense that the birth plan was a meaningful document that was read and understood by the staff who were looking after you?

C: It was very staff dependent. The plan is a set of preferences but that is absolutely not necessarily how your journey will go and, actually, just because you've read in a book that this might work well, I think it doesn't at all take into account the knowledge and skills of clinicians. I do worry about them, that they set women up who are going into labour this idea of what they are going to have and it's undeliverable. Nonetheless it's a statement of preferences that ought to be taken account of, even to the extent that people say, we know that you wanted this, it's in your birth plan but ...

When I got to the labour ward, I had a really good midwife there and she said, give me five minutes, I am just going to read through your birth plan. And she discussed it with me and she was like, yeah, we will try and take that into consideration as much as possible. The whole way through my birth plan I'd said, this is my idealised plan but I completely understand that circumstances change and would relish the opportunity to talk to a clinician about x, y and z if these circumstances change. So she definitely did listen to it.

So when I got up to the labour ward, the epidural situation happened and this really good midwife said, you definitely should have an epidural, reading your birth plan, and also I know how painful it is. She called the anaesthetist straightaway. Unfortunately it didn't work, the blood came out when it shouldn't, so they had to put in a second epidural. And then because they were worried about my son developing sepsis, they had to start the drug that speeds up labour. And unfortunately the epidural wasn't in correctly so the drug that brings about labour, it brings about really really painful strong contractions and unfortunately the epidural wasn't working, so I had ...

Was that just an error?

C: No, she was an incredibly senior anaesthetist and some people are just anatomically difficult, like it's really difficult to place them in some people. I was one of those people.

And you can't always tell that you have got it right until it's too late?

C: Exactly, until it's going. So she was absolutely excellent. My husband and I differ in our views on this. The reason I think that she was absolutely excellent was because she kept on coming back to check on me, calling in and saying, is the epidural right, it didn't seem like it was right. And she kept on coming to give me top-ups of medication into it to try and get it right. So she kept on coming back, she kept on asking me my opinion, and I think because I see with healthcare quite a lot of people do something and then walk away and it's impossible to get them back. I really really felt very looked after and unfortunately it didn't work.

We realised it wasn't working so she said, right, let's take it out, let's put another one in, so I had a third epidural. Unfortunately it worked apart from my left hip, here, so it was just really patchy. So when I've seen this in clinical practice, if you just top up with a bit more medication to go into the epidural then the patchiness clears up. So we tried to do that and I do worry that because I have a lot of knowledge about this then she possibly listened to me a little bit too much, because I said, oh no, I think if we top it up more I think it should go away, it's only a small area.

But because of my son's monitoring, they realised he wasn't doing so well, so they needed to top up the drug to speed up my labour. The pain just became absolutely unimaginable and I was screaming, I barely remember it. And the extreme pain on my body caused my baby's heart rate to drop and they had to put out an emergency call. So all the team ran in and I was so out of it that I didn't kind of realise what happened until everyone was there and trying to make decisions about whether I should be rushed for a caesarean to get the baby out. They decided to take the epidural out and put another one in – which also had a spinal in it as well, which is a slightly different type of pain relief – put both in together and instantly my pain just went. We didn't need to go for a caesarean straightaway so that I could try for another hour or so to see whether I would give birth naturally and if not consider having a caesarean at that point.

My husband feels that the anaesthetist botched putting the epidural in and that, had she done her job correctly, then none of that would have happened and we would have all been fine and ...

Is he a healthcare professional as well?

C: No. And I think that is probably the difference between my insight into how it can be and my husband's understanding. He could just see it didn't work so therefore she is bad at her job. Whereas I could see that she was incredibly diligent, worked incredibly hard at trying to make it work. Sometimes for some people it just doesn't work and it was really unfortunate that that person was me, but that wasn't through lack of effort. And she did say to me, I'm the most senior anaesthetist on, I'm very happy to get my junior to come and have a go ... if you would prefer somebody else to have a go at it. So she gave me opportunity to change the way things were going.

I've certainly seen plenty of epidurals in my practice that don't work and I've seen a lot of situations where people just go, it's fine, just top it up a little bit more, it will be fine, then walk away and leave the patient in agony. I see a lot of that in my time and that didn't happen for me.

What I think is, good care is probably more about the personal relationship that you have with that person, how diligent you are, how much effort you put in. I think of that as better care, whereas obviously I assume that if you are a senior, almost a consultant anaesthetist, then you have had your skill checked many a time. What matters to me most is how they make you feel and how well looked after you are.

So in the end I didn't progress at all, I'd been in labour for nearly forty hours. And I was only 4cm and you need to be 10. So I ended up going for a caesarean.

Can I ask a question? I mean, in retrospect, did they leave it too long before taking that decision, is it something that was foreseeable and maybe that decision should have been made at an earlier stage rather than leaving you forty hours in labour?

C: I think possibly. I think they work under the mantra that the less that they do is better, so there is a lot of post-op complications that you can get from having a caesarean, I got them all as well.

And so they tried to do as little as possible. And, actually, I was fine in the end, my son didn't develop sepsis – I mean, I had an awful time with pain relief, it wasn't anyone's real fault, so I think they probably judged it about right really. That opinion is probably formed as well having talked to some of my other friends in NCT [National Childbirth Trust], and two of them had another day on top of what I did and then had a caesarean at the end of it. So they had three-day-long labours, so actually I feel like I had a pretty easy ride, I think first-time babies do take a long time to come out. And also I had expected it would be horrendous, I think I just thought it would be awful and it was, so I think I went in with the idea that I wasn't going to be sitting listening to lovely music with candlelight and the baby just pops out …

So the caesarean was absolutely fine, it was better than I thought it would be, actually: it was quick, I felt very safe throughout the whole procedure, they talked to me, made me feel very comfortable. They did it under spinal, which is the medication that worked for me, but, yeah, they decided that they weren't sure about it because I'd had so many epidurals and spinals, it was quite unusual that he wanted to put a new spinal in, just to make sure that it definitely worked. So I think it was my fifth attempt – I know it wasn't ideal but I understood why. But I felt very reassured by all the machines and the drugs because that's what I'm used to, whereas other people would probably find it really unnerving …

After my operation, I went to the postnatal ward, which was like a living hell, to be honest. The ward was being built, there was a temporary ward and it was so hot, they had floor-to-ceiling windows but the blinds only went halfway down, so it was bright all the time. I think there were thirty-two beds and there were just curtains between all of them and so there was thirty-two screaming babies, everybody had a curtain round them, it was like a jail, it was tiny.

And suddenly you are launched into this area, I couldn't feel my legs because of my spinal, I'd just had a brand-new baby, I'd been in labour for forty hours, then had a major operation and … right, I'm going to do your observations, and then you are just left to get on with it. I thought that you would maybe get a little bit more tender loving care than, here's the baby you've got no idea what to do with, go for it. And I don't know exactly what it is that they could have done to make that less scary, but I certainly feel that there should be a step between you having a major operation and the postnatal ward, about one or two in the morning, feeling very drugged up and groggy and out of it. And then just being given a baby to look after, and I completely understand that that is what normally happens and I had been warned about it, but I just didn't feel that safe looking after him because I was just so exhausted.

Is the expectation that family members will be around?

C: Well, my husband was there, but equally he had been awake for forty hours as well. But they have very strict visiting rules, so actually you are not allowed any family members then at all; you are only allowed one extra person apart from your partner, at really strict times. Which I understand but I just didn't feel very safe looking after my son. I don't know what could be done differently about that but I feel after a normal operation you are very much looked after and they help you recover from that. With maternity, it feels like they forget that actually a caesarean is major abdominal surgery and you just get on with it. So it feels that there is a perception that because you have got a new baby, then it doesn't really matter that you have had a caesarean because it's so common.

I know that it's important to bond with the baby and have them next to you, it's crucial, but if you are so out of it you don't know whether you can put the baby back in the cot properly or you might fall asleep with the baby on you, which would be really unsafe … Maybe more staff, just somebody to sit with you for the first hour or two, I think that would make you feel so much safer.

How long were you there for?

C: Three days because you need to have some time there after your caesarean anyway but they were worried that my son had an infection. He had some infection markers in his blood, they needed to wait for some other blood results to come back and that took three days. And it was an absolute sweatbox, it was so hot, but they were really good there. I found it really hard to breastfeed at the start, very painful, and my milk hadn't come through and my baby was just screaming. And I was so glad of the midwives that were there. Again, it was that managing expectations and I saw a difference in the midwives' ability to do this. Some midwives just said, oh, you know, babies just cry, don't worry about it. Whereas there was this amazing midwife, she was clearly very experienced and she said, how old is he, I said day two nearly day three, and she said that is the worst possible time, the milk hasn't come through yet but it will come through by tomorrow morning. She said the next eight hours are going to be absolute hell but what we will do in the morning is, I will get you a breast pump and I will show you how to express and that will help your milk come through and then things will be better.

And she did and it was, and her giving me a plan – even though the next eight hours were horrendous, there was a light at the end of the tunnel and I could see how I was going to get out of that situation. And she was absolutely amazing, she was what made it bearable. And I don't know how people can be at home and have that experience, it must be awful. Because everyone goes through the same experience, basically the baby is just so upset because they need milk and your milk hasn't started coming out yet. Having somebody that's clearly knowledgeable, so much experience, had such a lovely manner, she was brilliant and had a plan.

It's the clinical competence along with the compassion, and one without the other doesn't work – it has to be both together. And I think that's what is wrong with a lot of healthcare: people can be very proficient at one or the other and it's those two together.

There were also healthcare assistants, they came round and did observations on myself and my son. I was able to call them and ask questions about how to look after my baby, can you help, he's crying and I don't know why. And when you ask them, they were clearly really busy but they were really good and they did help, they were fantastic. And they were very good at empowering me to look after my own child because they were very aware that you were going to be leaving sometime soon and you are going to have to do this by yourself. And no matter how many books you read about baby stuff, once baby is actually there, it's a very different situation.

And also I saw breastfeeding experts who came in; they gave absolutely conflicting advice. There were two of them, and it kind of became a bit of a running joke for my husband and I. One came in in the morning and one came in in the afternoon, I'd tell them my problem and one would say, you must feed off one breast at one time and not do the other one. And then the other one said that you had to do both each feed … So it was very little help really and it felt really frustrating, to be honest.

I saw doctors about once a day when they came on ward rounds. If there were any issues that developed, like a cold sore which I'd never had before, they said it's like the herpes virus, they were very worried that I might give that to my son, who had obviously an immature immune system. I didn't develop that in hospital – I must have already had the virus – but because I was so run down it flared up. They were really good at getting the experts to come in and see me. I definitely did think that the teams linked up well to deliver the care, even though it was incredibly busy. So they clearly had a very efficient machine in the postnatal ward ...

Then I went home and I went back in three times. Things with my son were absolutely fine, but on day five I moved him to his cot; I probably did more than I was supposed to. I was only moving my baby from there to there, my husband was having to do all of the lifting, and all of a sudden I just felt pop! and lots of warmth and looked down and the bed was covered in blood all over my shorts. I had a bleed from my caesarean wound so I had to go into hospital at five in the morning. That was quite frustrating, actually: they didn't believe me about how much blood had come out, they said, oh, no, it was just a little bit of wound juice ...

I'd taken a picture of my bathroom floor, which had blood everywhere and she said, no no, that would have just been from a little bit of fluid from your wound. I said it wasn't, it was blood. So they got the doctor to have a look at my wound and they took some bloods and sent me home and said to continue my antibiotics, which I had been on because I had sepsis. And then the next day they called me up and said, actually your blood results show that your haemoglobin level, which is red blood cells, it's very low. So I found that frustrating that I wasn't ... And I really don't like doing "because I'm a nurse, so I should know" kind of thing. I don't like doing that, so I pressed my point as much as I can without saying that, because I've had that done to me previously in healthcare and it's not nice, especially when it's an area for which you have no expertise. That said, I know what blood looks like and I know what a wound is. So, yeah, I felt frustrated about that.

Anyway, everything was going fine, I was doing my own wound dressings at home but I didn't get the feeling that there was a good plan, because I used to just ask for the stuff. I don't know what would have happened for somebody else who wasn't a nurse, whether they would have been given any training on how to do it or been given a district nurse referral. It was very much go on and get on with it. Which is fine because I could do it but there didn't seem to be a very linked-up service when you got out of the hospital. And also I think it was a bank holiday at the time so everything was a bit out of joint.

And then when the midwife came to see my wound on day ten, it still wasn't healing very well and looked infected, so she asked me to go back into the hospital. So I went back in and unfortunately I think I had to wait six or seven hours to see a doctor, who just said carry on with it and we will send you into clinic to have a look at it. I think they scanned it and they said there was a bit of a collection underneath but nothing to worry about too much ... but to carry on with my antibiotics. And then two days later, I was changing my dressing and there was an almighty pop and just loads of nasty stuff came out of my wound. Then about two hours later I just felt horrendous, I had a high temperature, I developed sepsis again.

So I ended up going back into hospital for another three days. Because I have got a penicillin allergy and I'd been on the frontline treatment for people with penicillin allergies since I'd left hospital, they were kind of at a loss as to what antibiotic to give to me. For a breast-feeding mum, there is loads that you can't have because it will affect the baby and I couldn't have any penicillin and I'd already had the other main one. So I ended up on really strong antibiotics, which did really affect my son. He was absolutely beside himself because his tummy, you could hear it going. So he basically didn't sleep for three days, I felt really really poorly and I think it was just exhaustion.

They were very good again at the sepsis management, they were very clinically efficient. As I was saying before, there is a one-hour timescale from when you diagnose someone with sepsis to start treatment and they did it all and they were fantastic and I was very well looked after. I went back to the horrible postnatal ward but they gave me a separate room this time because my baby was a little bit older, and so I didn't have loads of screaming new-borns, so that was really good ...

I got mastitis in both sides as well, so I had a wound infection and that. I was just generally really poorly. But I again felt listened to, they were very thorough, going through everything. I saw every specialist under the sun and they came in, they reviewed me, they talked to me appropriately. And I felt, even though I had a horrible time, that everything that could go wrong, did go wrong, I still feel that I had really good care because they got the right people in at the right time. It couldn't have been known that I would get mastitis and I'd get a wound infection in general. Obviously there was the time they didn't listen to me about the bleeding and things like that, but overall I do think I had good care. Which is probably a really damning indictment of how bad I think the care can be within the NHS, that I think of that catalogue of issues, that my over-arching feeling is that I did have good care. I don't know whether I have got low expectations or not.

Well, you are relating your experience and other people might have drawn different conclusions, but that's the conclusion that you drew.

C: Yeah. I think I'm just a realist and I know what it's like, I know what care I could have had in that situation and it was much better than I have seen care be. So I feel lucky.

It does raise the question whether somebody who is not a healthcare professional who had a similar experience would have thought they might have had bad care because so many things went wrong. Did you give feedback to the hospital about your experiences?

C: Yes, I did, and I also went in, they invited me in to see the consultant after, to go through and debrief everything that happened and go through it. It wasn't just because I was a healthcare professional, I think for anybody who has had a difficult time during labour or postnatally they do invite them back, and I found that very valuable. She took a lot of time to go through everything and asked if there was anything that I felt could have been improved on. So I was able to debrief in a very informal way, that actually the next time the anaesthetist was on shift that did all the epidurals, she came in to find me on the postnatal ward and asked if we could have a chat, and asked if we could go through what went wrong. Because she was saying that she'd been feeling absolutely dreadful about it, she couldn't get over it, it was clearly a situation that was out of the normal for her. I don't know whether she would have done that with everybody. I think she would, but it was good to know that she was using my experience to reflect on current practice and learn what could have changed and what could have been done differently. So I think that was excellent.

And my midwife who I really liked from my antenatal period, she was actually on holiday when I gave birth, but as soon as she got back, she emailed me and asked how everything had gone. And she asked if I wanted a formal debrief with her as well, which I didn't need, I was absolutely fine. But I definitely do feel that the maternity service really gave an opportunity to reflect on practice and look at where things went wrong. Whether they did anything with that information and did change anything, I am not sure.

Thinking back over the whole experience, what would you say were the learning points for the NHS, particularly in relation to maternity care, but maybe more generally as well?

C: Going through it chronologically, I'd say that having a named consistent midwife is incredibly reassuring, especially if you have gone through a traumatic event in early pregnancy, like I did. I found that absolutely invaluable and I think that even though I had an awful time at the start, I do think I had a good pregnancy apart from that. And I think that was in a big way due to the reassurance and guidance that that one midwife gave me. So I think, as much as they can, if they can have the same midwife, I think that would be fantastic.

In terms of my care in the hospital, when I said I didn't feel well and requested a set of observations, I think that's a realistic request. And if somebody says, I'm not feeling very well, do you mind doing my observations to check, I think that should be delivered. So I think that that should be reflected upon as to why that didn't happen.

I think that setting real expectations, be that of when you are going to deliver the next care, what's that going to look like, even if it's going to be bad, letting them know that. Knowing that has a huge impact upon how patients feel and there should be a huge effort to strive to do that.

I took a lot from the anaesthetist coming back and reflecting on what went wrong with me. If things had gone wrong in my practice, I will talk about it with my team but I never really go back to the patient themselves and talk to them about that, and I thought that was really valuable. And also made me feel good really, that she took the time out of her day to make sure that I was okay. So I think I would, in the future, if there was anything that went really wrong or I wasn't sure about, actually explore that not only with fellow healthcare professionals but the patient themselves. That's probably the thing I will change the most.

And they had an excellent sepsis trolley that I wanted to steal for my practice. It was this rolling six-stage what you need to do and all the equipment that you needed for sepsis management. I thought it was excellent. I have already texted my boss about that and said we should get one. So I saw things that were clinically better than in my area and have made changes.

It's essentially about having the clinical excellence and kindness to go with it. People understand that things go wrong and they get infections and that won't necessarily mean that they will think that they've had bad care, just as long as you explain why did that go wrong. It's the human factors that influence people's perception of their care, not actually the care itself sometimes.

Yes. And I think you can derive a lot of reassurance from seeing how the professionals react to something going wrong.

C: Definitely.

Judging whether something shouldn't have gone wrong is, I suppose, the more difficult one – whether it was avoidable.

C: Yeah. I think, I'm not sure if any of mine were avoidable. Everything that went wrong for me is not unexpected in labour and after in post-natal care; I just happened to have got most of them. And it's quite often the pattern that when one thing goes wrong, your body's unwell, so it's more likely for all the other things to go wrong, it's a bit of a domino effect really.

Story 2: James

James looked after his mum who had dementia for ten years (see Chapter 7, Story 23, pp. 187–192) and found himself becoming an older father, a year after his mother died. His partner was overdue with their first baby and had to be induced, which proved traumatic, and there were problems during and after the birth and in the following weeks. Two years later, James's partner gave birth to a second baby, which was also overdue. Having been called in, the parents endured a stressful wait of six days in hospital before the baby was induced.

James: I'm an older father. I spent almost ten years caring for my mother. My partner is quite a bit younger than me, she's 35 and I'm 53.

I did promise Mum that I would have grandchildren for her before she died, 'cause she really loved children. My partner was pushing me for it, but it was just impossible when I was doing that caring role. It was just absolutely impossible to think about having children while I was doing that. You think, well, what happens if I leave Mum, what's going to happen to her, she's going to go into care and she didn't want that. Thankfully, my partner was patient, and as soon as Mum passed away it was like, right, James, we're not messing about now.

And you've got two children?

J: Now I have. My little girl was born in 2018, literally a year after my mum died.

I'll be honest, caring for Mum was more difficult than caring for a baby. I think that was a good foundation course, looking after someone with dementia. A baby's a doddle because the baby just improves. With dementia and Alzheimer's, it declines.

We were hoping to have a home birth for the first and we had everything geared up for that pool at home. Then we went on these courses where they train you on doing it naturally and ... I felt like I was a bit of an old chap there because there were all these very young couples. I mean, some medium, but I was definitely the oldest dad in the playground there. But it didn't really matter. I just felt like I was more confident to ask questions about things and challenge things. I've no qualms about asking things, whereas when I was younger, I was quite shy and reserved. No one was judgemental about me at all. Which I have received, for example, from a library service ... When you take your children along to a toddler and baby group at a library, people assume that you're Grandad. I went grey when I was 30, but I've just lost a bit more of it. I just didn't say anything because I thought, I don't want to embarrass you in front of everyone else and I'll just take it.

So, it didn't all happen as planned with the water birth at home?

J: Not at all. My daughter was two weeks overdue. It was quite a traumatic birth. When she was induced, waters were broken. As soon as her waters were broken, my daughter's heart rate plummeted and then it was way up, so she had a floating heart baseline. The crash team had to come in about five or six times.

In the end she had an episiotomy. She did have significant blood loss. She had to have a blood transfusion. She lost 2 litres of blood. So it wasn't the sort of lovely home birth that you'd imagine; it was like the extreme opposite.

My partner was very stressed about it. It had quite a real effect on her, to the extent that after the birth and before the next birth we just had, she asked for a debrief. The matron came along to our house and she got them to talk through what actually happened.

One of the things that really stuck in my partner's mind, there was a comment made by a doctor at the time saying that oxytocin, the drug to bring on labour ... the doctor said, turn that down, it's a very dangerous drug. She was really frightened when that was said. It left quite a scar within. She was trying to work out: what really happened?

In the end the matron said that it was only a very low level of the drug that was being given anyway, quite late on in the process. So, it wasn't as big a deal as it sounded on the day and she was reassured by that.

I think they could have recognised how it affected my partner mentally better, or maybe there should have been a route for her to take to help her to put that to bed. She didn't have closure at all on it.

On to the postnatal period: my daughter was born on something like the ninetieth percentile – big baby, 9lb 8oz, two weeks overdue. Mum really wanted to breastfeed and she was really trying her best to breastfeed. It wasn't happening. Really struggled for the first two weeks. So we went out and bought all these things so she could ... She expressed and the baby started taking it off. But she lost loads of weight over two weeks, only just about within the permitted guidelines. It turns out that my daughter had a milk allergy. My partner virtually worked that out herself and stopped dairy herself and it solved it ... 'cause my daughter would be sick after every feed constantly, which was worrying, and she'd feed every twenty minutes because she was being sick constantly.

I think there's something there that needs to be looked at – an early recognition about this. Because she's now on the twenty-fifth percentile from the ninetieth. That's a significant drop, isn't it?

We were referred eventually to a dietitian and they put us on the milk ladder pathway, I think it is, for my daughter to gradually build up. So, take her off everything, which we'd already done, and then gradually build her up with a tolerance. Now she's great. It was very slow, and I think that my daughter suffered for quite a good few months before anything was done. I think there could be an improvement there in the testing for it or the diagnosis of it. The warning signs were there, weren't they?

So, in terms of child health beyond the first few months and all the surveillance, how's that been?

J: Fantastic. She's been very healthy. A couple of trips to the doctor, an infection and one round of antibiotics. She's been very healthy. My partner breastfed her for fourteen months...

We now get into the second pregnancy, and I suspect we might have a bit of anxiety about the birth?

J: Absolutely. In terms of the visits, et cetera, big baby, again, in the ninety-eighth percentile. The consultant there on one of the trips to the hospital made a comment that there's no way it's going to be a home birth, it's going to be labour ward at the hospital and that's it, you've no choice, really. My partner was quite annoyed about that because it took her choices away. 'Cause she's told that every birth is different, and just because things went a bit scary the first time, you can have a normal pregnancy and have a birth at home. The midwives are saying, well even though it's a big baby, it doesn't prevent you from having the baby at home. So, you're getting mixed messages there.

We took the view: let's have a really flexible plan, let's try and go for home if we can, if not, let's have the birth centre where you've got the nice pools, and if not, let's be really open-minded about the whole lot.

But my partner was a bit disappointed that consultant said that your only option is the labour ward. That's when she discussed that with the midwives, and the midwives had a meeting with the consultant … So, all the options are still on the table when it came to it, which is great.

Again, we went over the due date. The baby was due on the 28th of December and we got to 3rd January: we were to go in and be induced and have the waters broken, et cetera. So, once the waters are broken and she's induced, the birth centre went out the window, so it was on the labour ward. Which was fine, because it had a pool there. So, we went in on the 3rd of Jan., ready to go, all bags packed, childcare sorted out with my partner's mum, staying at her house while I could stay with my partner to support her.

We went in on the 3rd all geared up. Sorry, there's no beds, so you've got to stay on this ward here. Great, we had our own side room with a fold-down bed that I could sleep in there, but we had to be on call basically to get summoned in to have the waters broken. But what happens is people come in with emergency caesareans and their waters have already broken, so even though we were number one on the list to be seen and done, we were in there six days. I couldn't believe it – we were just sat there waiting.

It's like a conveyor belt. You've got the people on the ward waiting to go into the labour ward … and then the people on the labour ward have got to be cleared out to the postnatal ward, and there's no … My partner's mum said, when can I get back to work? I don't mind doing this [babysitting] for a short while, but this is six days. We're thinking, oh my goodness, what are we going to do? So luckily her aunty stepped in over the weekend to help. But it was quite stressful.

This is such a minor thing, but it matters. We're trying to get decent sleep during the night, ready to prepare for birth. You need that rest, don't you? My partner was on paracetamol, just a mild painkiller for her. She was woken up at four in the morning, just to take a paracetamol tablet, and you think, hang on a minute …

Did she feel able to say, please don't wake me?

J: She did do. But it should be an obvious thing. You let people get their rest and then they're more prepared and fit.

So anyway, the day came … twenty past four in the morning, bang, pack your stuff, we're off, straight off up to the labour ward. We got to the labour ward and thought, hang on a minute, there's loads of empty rooms here not being used: what's this about? The reality was there just weren't enough staff … It wasn't to do with the rooms at all, no, no. We had a student nurse who's followed my partner as part of her training development. Great, she's absolutely fantastic, and she was present at the birth. Fantastic. But the other lady, the other midwife, I think she'd been out for a couple of years working out in the field in the community, just booking in patients for visits. So she was quite rusty, shall we say, with all the equipment and everything. So it didn't instil a lot of confidence in me. But she was okay, fair play to her, but she was just a bit rusty on everything.

And you could tell: massive short-staffed. I'm thinking, right, we had all these issues with my daughter the first time, if this pans out the same way as my daughter did, I'm pretty scared about this. They broke the waters and, sure enough, my son's heart rate crashed, and we thought, oh no, here we go again. Thankfully, it came back up and levelled out so he had a stable baseline. That was it, it just happened once.

My partner was fab. They gave us an extra hour to give the natural process a chance to kick in. Sadly, it didn't kick in fast enough, so she had to have the hormone again, which accelerated it. Within two hours and five minutes of having that hormone, baby was there. Because he was so big, she started to tear slightly and she needed an extended episiotomy this time. The last ten minutes, baby's heart rate fell to Mum's heart rate, so they couldn't distinguish the difference. So they didn't know whether baby's heart rate was there or not.

So they said, right, we'll put like a little cord into his head and screw it in so we can measure baby's heart rate better. They put the cord in his head and said, right, we're going to switch the other monitor off and switch this monitor on that measures baby's heart rate. Switched it on, nothing. I just sort of looked at the student nurse and said, where's his heart rate? No one said a word. I just thought, oh my goodness, this last ten or twenty minutes you've not had a heartbeat for baby here. They went and got the sister, who came and said, oh right, yeah, I can find it. She put the other machine on and I can hear like a four or five beat difference between the two. Oh, can you hear that? That's impressive. Thankfully, it was there. But what had happened is they'd not connected the monitor properly to his head. But it was a scary moment. So of course my partner's stressing out, you know, But in the end, he came out. He was a whopper. He was 9lb 12oz, so he was another big one. He's been fab ever since.

I suppose my experience, it was a bit different than my partner's, because I saw it all while it was happening and panning out and I saw how professional … Especially the first birth with my daughter when we had the blood loss, how fantastic they worked as a team and how quickly … to get the transfusion and everything and to bring the womb down in size. It was so professional and slick and I had total confidence in them that first time.

Whereas all my partner's memory was that doctor that said, this is a very dangerous drug, turn it down, turn it down. For me, I've been trying to give my perspective on it, but her perspective was tarnished by that thing happening.

With my son, everything's been fine since. But he's started to be sick now. It could be the same thing, milk intolerance. My partner's cut dairy out. But with my daughter she lost that huge amount of weight initially. My son has just put it on and on and on, so he's ... getting what he needs.

After the birth, it took two hours to stitch my partner back together. So, when we were back home, it's quite full-on for me 'cause my partner was in bed, she had trouble getting in and out of bed, we had my daughter running around. But it's fine. We got through that first couple of weeks, which were quite tough, and then, of course, I'm back to work straightaway. So, from a dad's perspective, it was a full-on two weeks. Thank goodness you get paternity leave. It was really not a time to enjoy the baby ... shopping, sort my daughter out, cooking, cleaning, make sure my partner's all right. So, it's not the dream that you have in your mind, just sat there with baby on your chest, bonding.

Being included by the NHS, well, it's helped me support my partner more, I think, and it's given me confidence. Even though everything's not perfect, is it? I've had to try and absorb my partner's stresses and concerns and manage them, I feel, but that's part of being a partner, isn't it?

PREGNANCY AND CHILDBIRTH: REFLECTIONS AND RESPONSES TO THESE STORIES

Immediate questions

1. Why was continuity of care important to Cathy during her pregnancy?
2. To what extent do you agree with Cathy's overall assessment of the quality of care she received?
3. What do both Cathy's and James's experiences tell us about the importance of managing expectations?
4. In what ways was Cathy's professional nursing experience both a help and a hindrance?

5. Should James's partner have been given more choice over the manner of her second birth? How could this issue have been differently handled?
6. What do James's and Cathy's stories suggest about good practice in how healthcare professionals communicate with partners?

Strategic questions
1. What changes in maternity services policies would improve the experience for mothers and their partners?
2. How can frontline professionals be better equipped and enabled to support women in pregnancy and childbirth?
3. What do you think are the organisational cultural barriers to person-centred maternity care? How can these be overcome?
4. What actions can you take as a policymaker, professional leader, frontline member of staff or NHS manager to improve the experience of care for mothers and their partners?

REFERENCES

Department of Health (1993) *Changing Childbirth, Part I: Report of the expert maternity group* (London: HMSO).

Knight, M., K. Bunch, D. Tuffnell, J. Shakespeare, R. Kotnis, S. Kenyon and J.J. Kurinczuk (2019) *Saving Lives, Improving Mothers' Care: Lessons learned to inform maternity care from the UK and Ireland Confidential Enquiries into maternal deaths and morbidity 2015–17* (Oxford: National Perinatal Epidemiology Unit, University of Oxford).

Mellor, J. and N. Chambers (1995) "Addressing the patient's agenda in the reorganisation of antenatal and infant health care: experience in one general practice", *British Journal of General Practice* 45: 423–425.

Morecambe Bay Investigation (2015) *Report*, www.gov.uk/government/publications/morecambe-bay-investigation-report (accessed 25 March 2021).

NHS England (2016) *National Maternity Review Report: Improving outcomes of maternity services in England*, www.england.nhs.uk/wp-content/uploads/2016/02/national-maternity-review-report.pdf (accessed 5 January 2021).

Ockenden Report (2020) *Emerging Findings and Recommendations from the Independent Review of Maternity Services at the Shrewsbury and Telford*

Hospital NHS Trust, HC 1081 (London: Department of Health and Social Care), https://www.gov.uk/government/publications/ockenden-review-of-maternity-services-at-shrewsbury-and-telford-hospital-nhs-trust (accessed 25 March 2021).

Petersen E.E., N.L. Davis, D. Goodman et al. (2019) "Racial/ethnic disparities in pregnancy-related deaths – United States, 2007–2016", *MMWR Morbidity and Mortality Weekly Report* 68: 762–765.

✷ 3 ✷

CHILDREN AND YOUNG PEOPLE

INTRODUCTION

Children and young people are not just smaller adults. Their bodies and minds, and associated health and care needs, are different and distinct, requiring a dedicated, expert and age-sensitive approach. The English health and care system is not fully adapted to this reality. Though the role of paediatricians is generally prized and at its best ensures a personalised, age-appropriate, child-centred and holistic approach to secondary medical care, overall quality is variable. In the UK, health visitors focus on prevention and support for parents of 0–5-year-olds, which is a cornerstone of World Health Organization (WHO) primary healthcare policy (WHO, 2008). The people who work in this service have recently experienced a significant drop in numbers, restrictions in mandatory scope, policy flux in relation to their role, and structural distancing from their family doctor colleagues, to the extent that one GP recently said that health visitors were "out there somewhere", but exactly where was a mystery to him (Bryar et al., 2017).

The NHS Long Term Plan in England (NHS, 2019) acknowledges improvements in some services in England but gives a mixed picture overall. A number of child health outcomes lag behind those in other comparable countries (though social and economic factors such as poverty and deprivation play an important part in this too). There are particular problems with mental ill health, mortality (including neonatal deaths and deaths from respiratory conditions such as asthma) and obesity. Children from deprived areas or with a black or minority ethnic family background are twice as likely to be obese as those from other backgrounds, and this inequality is widening (Public Health England, 2018).

Children with complex needs and disabilities are often under-served, with parents struggling to access help and support for their children, especially from local authority social services and education departments, and to achieve coordination between different services (Council for Disabled Children, 2019). Anxious and exhausted parents often find that the system does not respond well to their own needs as carers (Smith et al., 2015). The transition from child to adult services can be fraught and lead to discontinuities of care (Colver et al., 2019).

In recent years there has been growing awareness and concern about the level of mental ill health among children and young people and the extent to which the NHS is able to cope (King's Fund, 2017). A survey of young people published in 2019 by the Royal College of Paediatrics and Child Health highlighted calls for quicker referrals, better staff training, better mental health support, more focus on equipping young people with self-care skills, and closer listening to young people in decisions about individual care and services (Royal College of Paediatrics and Child Health, 2019). Under the Long Term Plan, the NHS has committed to improvements in child health services across a broad front, including more integrated services, the move to a 0–25-year service and better provision for young people with autism and learning disabilities.

THE STORIES

As with the other chapters, we invite you, the reader, to immerse yourself in the stories and then reflect. In Chapter 1 (Section 2, p. 4) we offer an understanding of patient-centred care in general as:

- Understanding and valuing what matters to patients
- Seeing the whole person
- Respecting people's rights and autonomy
- Being customer focussed

At the end of the chapter, we have posed a few questions arising from the following stories. We have tried to do this in such a way to provoke rather than to constrain your own thinking. As a patient or carer, a healthcare professional, an NHS manager or anyone else with an interest in child health, what issues are raised by these testimonies? What can be done and what can you do to improve the way that care can be organised around children and young people – and their carers?

Four contrasting stories are presented here. **Dan** is a normally healthy teenager who was hospitalised with an acute bacterial infection from which he has now recovered. His father Jonathan tells the story from his perspective. Dan's illness took place during the COVID-19 pandemic, and some of the features of his care and treatment reflect changes to NHS services which were necessitated by the pandemic. **Jim** was a severely disabled young man from birth until his death aged 36. His parents Justin and Lucinda cover his entire life – and death – in their account. In a story fragment, **Eve** remembers how as a child she came to be diagnosed with Type 1 diabetes. Finally, the story of **Finbar** is related by his mother, who tells of her experiences as a carer for her teenage son with a diagnosis of scoliosis, including the length of time taken to get an appropriate tertiary referral, and the need to track and chivvy to get appointments and get the operation scheduled. Her experience of a support group was very helpful to her.

Story 3: Dan and Jonathan

16-year-old Dan began complaining of back ache one Friday evening following a bike ride during the COVID-19 lockdown. The symptoms worsened over the next several days, with Dan suffering pain, loss of mobility, poor sleep, swollen joints and eventually jaundice. His father Jonathan sought help from NHS 111 and the local GP surgery. Though he was impressed by the swift response of both services – Dan was prescribed powerful pain and sleeping medication – these did not seem to be working. A week after the initial onset of symptoms, Jonathan made a repeat phone call to the local surgery and a GP asked him to bring Dan in. There were many examples of care and kindness. At times Dan's parents were overwhelmed by the amount of information they were given, and it was not always clear who was in charge on the ward.

Jonathan: So we went in and we were the only patients there and I couldn't help noticing how bizarre it all was to go into a GP surgery where there is no one there and then the GP saw us and he had, you know, enough time to do a thorough investigation. He didn't know what it was. And he said, "I want to book you in for some blood tests." And he said, "In the meantime if it gets worse and you are really worried, go straight to A&E." And he said, "Don't worry about going to A&E during lockdown because this doesn't look like COVID so you'll go to a non-COVID part and actually they're really quiet up there." In fact – and he made a bit of a joke about this – "they are dying to see people, they'd love it if you turned up." We had a bit of laugh about it because this seemed so bizarre for any doctors kicking their heels waiting for patients to turn up.

On the Sunday, still worried, Jonathan did take Dan to A&E. It was very quiet and they were seen immediately. Tests were done and in the absence of a definitive diagnosis Dan was admitted to the paediatric department, where he spent the next three weeks. During the first few days:

J: We were sort of bombarded with information and tests and investigations. It was quite a bewildering and anxious time. He was in the care of the paediatric department. He also came under the attention of the orthopaedic department because of all the joint pain and mobility issues. He came under the attention of the cardiologists because they were worried that he had a bacterial infection that could get to the lining of the heart and cause something called infective endocarditis. And also the infectious diseases department. And then during that period also they did some scans and so the radiologists were involved and they found a big abscess on a muscle and they then operated on it. During that time they found he had a bacterial infection – a staphylococcus aureus infection – they thought it had caused the abscesses. They didn't know whether other things were going on as well, they couldn't quite explain the jaundice. They thought that might have been caused by all the medication he had been on.

An added complication was the COVID-19 pandemic.

J: They also did a COVID test on him. In order to do that they took him and put him in a different ward in the COVID section of the hospital, which alarmed my wife – well, we were all alarmed because we couldn't see the logic of it. My wife tells a story about how she sat in a chair to stop people coming in because she was worried about COVID infection and she was paranoid about it and she couldn't understand why she hadn't been tested even though Dan had been tested. And he was there I think for about forty-eight hours until he got the all clear and then he went back to his previous bed in the paediatric ward. It was all very weird: the parents were never tested and we could come and go, and so the COVID procedures seemed to be somewhat haphazard.

Then I said to my wife, "Look this is mad, you need to come home and have a rest." And from then on we did a rota so that we alternated every twenty-four hours and so one of us was there overnight. The first week was the most alarming because they put him on antibiotics, a very high dose. What they said was ... of course we were Googling like mad as you do ... but the most dangerous thing that could happen really would be an infection of the heart lining and that could be fatal, so they were zapping him with antibiotics. Then they made a decision that they could reduce the dosage and over that week, they became less worried about his heart but they were still worried about the fact that it was taking a long time to kill off the infection and so he had daily bloods, and the level of infection was going down but it hadn't been eliminated and what they said was they want to kill it off completely and from the point that it's a negative test, they then want to give him two weeks of intravenous antibiotics and then they can send him home and he has four weeks of antibiotics taken orally. So in other words, they were taking absolutely no chances with this bug.

In the first few days Dan was bedbound and needed a lot of hands-on care.

J: This was one of the reasons why we felt instinctively that we had to be there. He got very hot, he needed to be rolled over, he needed to be fanned, and in fact we had to bring in a fan as they didn't have one. He needed cold towel washes. The other big part of the first two weeks was draining the abscess and having this tube hanging out into a bag while it continued to drain for several days. When we rolled him over we had to keep making sure that we weren't trapping the tube that was draining from his upper thigh into this bloody horrible bag.

Also, he needed to wee into a bottle and have it emptied. One of the weird things was that we know him as a fully post-pubescent 16-year-old, 6 foot 6 boy, who in normal circumstances, would totally, you know, protect his privacy and dignity. Lying there naked because it was too hot to wear clothes and he hated the hospital gown, I would sort of try and look away as he was weeing into his bottle and then he would say, "Yeah, forget it, Dad, it's okay, my dignity has gone out of the window, it doesn't really matter now," and he was really quite cool about it.

Supposing you hadn't been there, what would've happened? I assume he would have had to call the nurse or somebody?

J: We would have been very worried about him and whether he was getting the care that he needed. As it was, he was calling them quite a lot. The IV machine would beep all the time, it would beep to warn you it was going to end and it beeped when it did end. Or it beeped because it said there was a blockage. So quite a lot of time was spent calling the nurses to come and turn the machine off or fix the problem or, you know the infusion is ended. One of the things we learned was, when the infusion is ended, it's fine, you are not going to suddenly get pumped full of air in your veins and die of an embolism. It took a while before we got a proper explanation and we still worried about it as occasionally air bubbles would appear. And we'd think, "Is this serious, should I call the nurse?" It's funny, Dan was quite happy to call the nurses and be a demanding patient. Whereas I often felt that I didn't want to disturb the nurses, so he was quite a good advocate for himself – probably better than I was.

Interesting. Why do you think there was that difference?

J: Oh, he's a teenager, lacks deference. He was very charming, he's got quite a way about him. He was completely unabashed about calling for help. The nurses really liked him but he was calling them all the time. That could have been reduced if instead of having a machine that beeps by the ear of the patient and their worried parent, you had a machine that alerts the nurse in the place where the nurse is.

The family had to digest a huge amount of information.

J: One of the issues was there's an awful lot of information to absorb. We saw the orthopods and the paediatricians and the radiologists quite a lot. They were very good at doing their best to convey lots of information about what they thought was happening, what the treatment plan was and what was going to happen next. It was very patient-centred and very parent-centred. But it was very difficult to make sense of. Both Marianne and myself were taking notes just in order that we could go back and look at what was being said if there were any problems later. It's not because we didn't trust them. There was almost too much information. I mean, we probably didn't help by asking lots of questions and trying to make sense of it all. Their willingness to explain, I thought, was really good, I couldn't fault it. But it was all quite confusing.

Did Dan say he thought it was a bit much as well?

J: Yes, at one point, he did say, "There's just too much information." And it may be partly because they were always talking in the presence of Dan and he's a minor and so they are probably thinking that I need to explain this quite thoroughly and carefully to somebody who is a child. So they maybe could have done more checking on information needs; I think that's a more sophisticated approach.

So, after the first week of anxiety, we got the news that the germ had been killed off and the blood cultures were negative. That was a big turning point and we were able to relax. It was only at that point, where I think the paediatrician said, "Actually we've been quite worried about how long it took to kill off the infection, it normally takes forty-eight hours and this took about a week." And so they hadn't shared all their worries with us and actually I was glad as we had enough worries.

Can I ask about that? The received wisdom is that you shouldn't hold back from sharing with family what's going on, but on this occasion you felt this was the right call?

J: Well, it was in a context of relief that things were okay. My thought was, well, actually I'm quite glad that you didn't burden me with that extra worry as I was worried enough already. It's not as if they weren't telling us quite a lot. So, yes, it made me reflect on my own need for timely and accurate information. You have to make a judgement about it, I think, based on what you think the expectations of a parent are.

Dan was delighted by unexpected visits from the A&E staff.

J: At various times, all three of the clinicians who had been on duty when Dan came into A&E – the nurse, the consultant and the junior doctor – came up to visit. And of course it was very quiet in A&E but nonetheless, the fact that they'd made the effort was absolutely lovely. It was just a spontaneous demonstration of caring. They didn't have to.

Do you think there's also an element, because they were quieter because of COVID-19, there was a kind of medical curiosity as to what was going on with that?

J: I'm sure they were curious because he was an interesting case. I don't mind that.

How did Dan react when they came up and said how are you getting on?

J: Ah, he was overjoyed. He was really chuffed and he liked them, they all had a really good rapport. This is paediatric A&E, so I guess they are predisposed and selected on the basis that they are good at relating to young people. But they were … all three of them were just really nice.

Can you tell me how important that was for you and Marianne and for Dan that they did that, made that journey from the first to the seventh floor?

J: There was just something about the sense that he'd been remembered. It said something about continuity, about people aren't just looking after you because you've ended up in their patch, they actually think about you when you're not there, and come and seek you out. It's not something that you'd expect or demand as a matter of course. Indeed, in most cases it just wouldn't be practical, but it was just a lovely bonus.

Though Jonathan's assessment of Dan's care and treatment is overall very positive, there were a number of irritating aspects.

J: People were always asking him how tall he was. A paediatric patient of 6 foot 6 is a bit of rarity and I think people were curious and enjoying his rarity value but he got a bit bored … actually he did get a bit fed up with that. Strictly speaking, you know, when everybody's doing it, it starts to feel as though people aren't respecting you.

It's quite insensitive, actually. It could be perceived as that after a while.

J: I think he took it in good part and it wasn't such a big deal for him but I think from time to time I got the sense that he found it slightly irritating. People can be sensitive about their height, not all tall people enjoy being tall. Actually he's fine with it but, you know, people have all kinds of body issues. How could they know he wasn't sensitive about his height? So for me that felt a bit off.

Jonathan has a number of observations about the nursing.

J: The nursing staff were interesting because it was actually quite difficult to work out what status and authority the different nurses had. I think there is a colour coding in the uniforms. It was never clear. There was never the equivalent of what the consultants did. They would tend to introduce themselves and say, "Hi, I'm a consultant this and I'm a consultant that and my name is so and so." Whereas the nurses would tend to introduce themselves by their first names and say, "Hi, I'm so and so and I'm on duty tonight," but it wasn't always clear how senior they were and how much authority they had. You want to know who's in charge.
  In the entire time we were there, which was three weeks, we encountered one senior nurse in the "classic" style, which people of my age are

used to. She was of a certain age, she must have been in her late 40s or early 50s, and she had a very authoritative manner, she told you exactly what was going to happen and exactly what she was going to do, and she went about things in a brisk and efficient way and created waves of calm and reassurance around her. Whereas most of the nurses seemed fresh out of college, they all seemed so incredibly young and it just wasn't clear how much skill and experience they had.

And from time to time, you did wonder when they, for example, fumbled with taking blood or fumbled with changing a cannula ... Almost comically, because Dan had this huge abscess on one of his toes (a bizarre thing) which then got drained painfully and then needed to be dressed, the only people who seemed to be able to dress this damn toe were the orthopaedic doctors, but they had this habit of coming along and undoing the dressing every time they investigated it to check how it was doing and then leaving it undressed and then assuming that a nurse would do the dressing.

Then generally speaking, a nurse wouldn't do the dressing unless we'd ask and some nurse would do the dressing and it would fall off again. It became a point of comedy between us about how rubbish the nurses were at doing dressings. Particularly as Dan got out of bed and started to mobilise, the first thing that would happen was his toe dressing would fall off.

I think, how hard can it be, isn't that basic nursing? What is going on here? I can't think of a nurse who wasn't kind and caring. But they weren't always good at the basics, and the other basic thing was that sometimes Dan was in a lot of pain and needed pain relief. You know, we just wanted it to be delivered quickly and not to have to go and pester the nurses for it.

Jonathan also reflected on the difference in status and authority as between the nurses and doctors.

J: The doctors were the ones with daily visits and daily information, often with the results of blood tests that had been done the previous day. They came with revised treatment plans or confirmed treatment plans and the sense that we got was that the doctors are in charge and the role of the nurses implicitly was one to just execute whatever decisions the doctors had made. There was no sense that the nurses had any independent authority to do anything in particular. Even though they may have done, that was never clear to us. The doctors are the people who turn up when they turn up and you have no means of getting hold of them. They turn up on their ward rounds and they tell you stuff. The nurses are the people you can call with your buttons, so they are like servants who can be called. It's very interesting how the work practice and the design layout also send messages about who is charge.

The doctors come in their own time. The nurses, at least in theory, are there to be called in your time although they don't always respond in the time that you want. But it is interesting how that sends a signal, doesn't it, about the relative status of doctors and nurses.

And a final reflection on the intravenous infusion pump:

J: The bleeps are noisy and intrusive and can be alarming and they are not heard by the nurse so you always have to call a nurse to turn the machine off. And if you know you are infusing somebody you'll know how long it lasts because the machine is programmed to do it for thirty minutes; even if you can't hear it, then you should be back in thirty minutes in time to turn it off. In practice, the nurses needed to be called and I am happy to give them the benefit of the doubt that it was because they were busy with other patients. In which case the problem was a technical one, which is if you've got a machine that is going to send reminders to people that they need to take some action then the reminder needs to be directed to the person who needs to be reminded, which is not the patient and not the carer, who are not in a position to do anything about it and it may just make them more anxious.

Story 4: Jim, Lucinda and Justin

Jim had physical and learning disabilities from birth, and associated health and behavioural problems. He was diagnosed with Robinow syndrome, a rare genetic disorder. He lived with his parents Justin and Lucinda until his death aged 36. He also had a younger sister Rosemary. His parents explored residential care options for Jim when he was younger but decided that having him at home was the best option. During his life he and his parents had many interactions with NHS and social care services. His parents spoke about Jim a few months after his death.

Lucinda: When Jim was born I didn't think anything was wrong. Before he was born I had a scan and I read the results (I shouldn't have done but I did) and it said that the baby had a big head. And when I went down to see the doctor to share the scan, I mentioned that and he said, "Oh, babies' heads are different shapes, lots of babies have big heads," and so I didn't really think it was going to be a problem. When Jim was born, he was born very quickly. I didn't have time for any drugs at all and he was very small and of course I didn't realise anything was wrong except everyone's faces and an air of panic in the room. When Jim was delivered we thought we had a little girl and when I held him I realised there was something dreadfully wrong. He had an enormous head and a tiny, tiny body.

And we went to a normal ward and everyone was having visitors and celebrating having a baby and I got very upset and asked if I could be moved. And then they provided a side ward and I went on my own. And then a very good young doctor came, a lady, and she was lovely. We had a consultant. He did lots of tests, but straightaway he said that this child isn't Downs because you can see the lines of his palms. And I only saw him the once, I think. Over the next few days we had another consultant called Dr X, who was our consultant for over eighteen years, I think.

That was great. We used to visit him in XXX and he was very supportive, did lots of research.

Justin: At that time you had to bear in mind that the number of documented cases of his syndrome were very, very few indeed and were in America. So information was difficult to come by as it was pre-Internet. There are many, many more documented cases now than there were. They're mostly in America and he's not typical in any case because he has other issues that are not specific to Robinow syndrome, which is what he had, having been the name of the person who identified it initially.

It's worth mentioning here his genitalia was not specific. In other words, it looked as if his penis was more like a clitoris than a penis and he had no testes as well; there was no evidence of a scrotum and so on. So it was difficult.

So Dr X provided that care and support over eighteen years?

J: Until Jim stopped being a child effectively and became an adult.

What difference did that make to you?

L: Huge difference. He was just a very kind person.
J: He wasn't a specialist other than the fact he was a paediatrician. He wasn't particularly familiar with children with disabilities. He'd obviously had children under his care that had disabilities but that wasn't his specific specialism, as far as I know.

And that didn't bother you, that wasn't particularly important to you?

J: It was such a rare syndrome there wouldn't have been anybody like that available in any case, certainly not locally. I mean, the prognosis about his life generally at that stage wasn't particularly good in any case. I think twice we were called to XXX as they said, "You'd better come to the hospital straightaway," and he pulled through.

In terms of social workers, I don't know where to start, really, with that because, over the years we had a whole stream of different people; they didn't seem to stay with the service very long, some were better than others and some were completely useless.

L: I think we were fortunate because we were transferred to XXX maternity home. It was a very small unit and I think there were three of us on the ward and you could stay on the ward as long as you wanted to, pretty much. And that was lovely because at that point Jim was having tests to see his gender. We were told that we could decide if we wanted him to be a girl or boy. The staff there, I remember, the nurses were very supportive and they were very kind. Do you remember, Justin?

We decided that he'd be a boy and it was all a bit confusing for people because we'd said we'd had a girl. I don't know how we got round that. The medical practice in XXX were really good, GPs would come out if we needed.

J: Of course the GPs would come out to you in any case at that time. It was that era. And Dr X was a very kind and gentle person.

The GPs and paediatricians didn't know much about Robinow syndrome, but that didn't matter particularly did it, I guess?

J: No, because any problems that he had were not related to the typical case of Robinow syndrome. There were other issues that he had. He had breathing difficulties, he had a restricted oesophagus and windpipe. He had issues with swallowing and breathing. It could have been anybody, really.

Jim spent much time in hospital as a child. The care was mostly good but his parents describe one bad incident.

L: Yes, it was in the children's hospital, actually, and Jim had a hernia when he was quite small. We went into the room and the doctor that was going to do it asked if he could bring some students in and I said yes. And then they took Jim's pad off and he said to them, "You've never seen anything like this before and you never will again."

J: And you were upset. People engaging mouth before engaging brain about the impact it's going to have. It's all right saying that to students, but when the mother's there as well, it was a bit unthinking, wasn't it?

Was there any sense from looking at his face or those of the students that they had an understanding of that impact?

L: Yeah, I think the students did. I don't think he did. They were embarrassed.

Lucinda and Justin describe Jim's health problems and disabilities.

J: He had some mobility issues which were ongoing. I mean, over the years he could walk better if he was inclined to do so. He was only the same size of a 9-year-old. So he was small in stature. The other difficulties were feeding. Initially he would have everything done for him but he did get to the point at one stage where he would drink from a bottle with a teat on. But then we were advised not to do that by the health visitor, because we were giving him sugary drinks and that could give him tooth decay over a period of time, blah-de-blah. He had difficulty swallowing because his oesophagus was constricted and so the food had to be chopped up very small. And this got worse as the time went on. I mean, naturally we had to blend all his food to soup-like consistency. That was partly due to the restriction in his tubes but also because he developed a problem with acid indigestion, acid reflux. The stomach valve didn't work properly and so he'd get food coming back up and an acid which burnt his throat. And then, obviously, it was a bit of a vicious circle because he didn't want to eat as it hurt to swallow.

So we went to see a gastro specialist in XXX and the first one was useless, wasn't he? He said had we tried doing, this, that and the other. He was just very unkind. He said, "He might be bringing stuff up because you are making him swallow it too much at a time." There was all sorts of things. Anyway, in the end, we did actually say to the hospital could we see someone else and we saw somebody who was much more sympathetic.

Well, he prescribed some medication to help with the reflux, which he was on until he died. But that situation got worse and worse and he would vomit, especially if he was lying down. He was less likely to vomit when he was vertical than when he was horizontal. So we had to keep his head raised in bed eventually and things like that. I mean, we got up – I don't know – innumerable times we had to get up in the night, sometimes two or three times in the night to go and change him and his bedclothes because he'd vomited. This was all due to this acid reflux band so the drugs were only partially effective. He was always having problems with lumps in his food, you know, we had choking incidents in the past when I've had to do a Heimlich or turn him upside down and pat his back and stuff.

And he had speech and language difficulties, didn't he?

L: No speech at all.

J: He understood a lot more than he could convey to you. The noises he made would give you an indication of his moods. He could laugh, he could cry and those types of emotions. He could express pain but there was nothing we would call intelligent about the noises that he made unless you understood him like we do.

L: He was doubly incontinent.

J: Oh yes, there was all that. Right the way through his life. We did try to train him to use the toilet but it wasn't possible. We tried and tried and we just had to give up in the end.

L: At the end of his life, we seemed to have lots of therapists. We had a speech therapist. What else did he have, Justin? He was partly deaf in one ear, more than he was in the other …

J: We saw somebody that was organised by that nice speech therapist who told us why he couldn't drink from a beaker and things which no one had ever told us before. Because he had problems with his jaw. His bottom teeth overshot his top teeth, which made chewing difficult and it also made drinking difficult. We never realised why he was so reluctant to drink other than from a spoon. We had at least two speech therapists before that. And also we got advice about feeding from the speech and language therapist department as well. Some of which was better than others, you know. You don't know until you try these things.

Justin and Lucinda describe the problems of hospital admissions once Jim had become 18.

L: That brought its own problems because then we had to go into mainstream hospital and he'd be on a ward with adults, which was awful. It was at Christmas, Christmas morning, and he'd had gastroenteritis and he was rushed in and he was taken into an adult ward. I got so cross because they really were not looking after him, expecting me to do everything, and I was in a state and you just wanted a bit of help and advice, really. I remember being very upset about that.

J: Throughout, it's always been a struggle because every professional that has had any dealings with us, and with Jim, treat him as his real chronological age. There was no allowance made for the fact he was still basically a child. All his life he was a child. He never progressed from being a child mentally. And physically he looked like a child with his stature being so small. That has been an issue time and time again.

Later experiences in other hospitals were better. Over the decades, Justin and Lucinda felt that the hospitals improved their understanding about how to deal with disability. They reflect on a particularly good social worker.

J: There was that scatter-brained woman who used to spill her handbag all over the floor.
L: Yes, she was good. She seemed to understand Jim and understand us I think. You got to know her well … When you have lots of social workers, every time they come it's a formal meeting, you are repeating yourself, and other times they ask you the same …
J: You fill out the same form, you say the same thing.
L: And then you take Jim off to the centre so that they can meet him and they say, "We've seen Jim now, okay," and tick a box. But she always sat with Jim.
J: She interacted with him.

Justin and Lucinda describe the difficulties in obtaining respite care.

J: One of the issues was the fact that there was a lot of change in staff. There wouldn't be the same people there every time you went in and so therefore there was not always the understanding of his particular needs that perhaps there should have been. There were issues about if he was poorly, he would be immediately hospitalised, even if we were away on holiday, and then some member of staff would have to go with him and then they couldn't stay, as they were short of staff. I worried … Rosemary [Jim's sister] had helped out quite a bit in that respect but obviously she has her own children and she's got her own job and so on, she works. On one occasion they insisted … I had to fly back from Ibiza, was it? I had to go and sit with him in hospital for three days and then when it looked as though he was recovered I went back out. Now, that wasn't an issue as I was probably the best person to be with him and help him, in terms of the fact when he once started to take fluids he perked up a lot. But they said: "… well, it's not our job. If people are ill it's not our job to look after them …" Well, what good is respite if you can't go on holiday? That wasn't the first time. We were constantly on edge and Lucinda would say to me, "Ring up and check he's all right." And I know damn well I'd get a phone call if he wasn't. You know, really your whole life was dominated by caring anyway, and if the respite service couldn't provide you with respite if he was not feeling well, then it wasn't luxurious was it?

The other thing was that we had, through social services, arranged something called "adult placement". There was a guy who was really good about finding people who would take Jim over a weekend or a few days or just for one night or if something cropped up at short notice like you want to go to a funeral or something like that, he got somewhere where he could go. And then we went through one or two, lots of people, but it didn't last long, most of them. They found somebody in XXX and she was excellent. You had other adults there and it got very difficult because Jim would get up in the night and start wandering about and disturb the other service users and so on. She was brilliant. Then social services, they stopped ... they said they couldn't divide the respite care between two lots of services. So adult placement and the county council provided respite. I couldn't understand why somebody like the social worker couldn't monitor how many hours or days or whatever they had in the one place. And then the social worker said, "I shouldn't rock the boat if I was you as very few people get the amount of time that you get" – yes, quite. So it sort of petered out, didn't it, the placement?

There was no continuity of staff. There weren't always the same people around when Jim was there. We had issues about the levels of personal hygiene, as he always got sick when he came back from there. You know you've got people who don't understand personal hygiene being there with him.

L: You mean service users, not the staff.

J: Other service users, yeah, who didn't understand personal hygiene because they've all got learning difficulties and so very often he would get sick or soon after he came back from there.

Justin and Lucinda talk about Jim's behavioural issues and the impact on their own health of caring for Jim.

J: When he was younger it was quite difficult to go anywhere. You had to be very aware of what he was doing as he could lash out and smash ornaments and things like that. I think he broke two televisions in our house ... he used to have a TV in his room ... until I managed to get a means of screwing them to the wall. I think ... he has frustration, or perhaps not being able to express if he was in pain. But just general frustration at not being able to express himself. In terms of help with that, he was prescribed with ... what was that drug? It was a sedative-type drug to calm him down anyway. We did try it. One tablet was far too much as it just knocked him out and then it broke his routine. It messed with his sleep pattern. And even half a tablet had an impact which we thought was undesirable. At one time we asked the doctor about sleeping pills and he said, "Well, they don't really work unless you … you have to know that you've taken them", sort of thing. I don't know, well, anyway. Usually the tablets went out of date before he ever took them. But they were there and they used to go with him to respite. I don't know that they ever used them.

L: I don't think they did. The pills just wiped him out. He'd be asleep for the next day, all day. It was horrible.

J: It was horrible. So rather than that, we just put up with him with it. He would pull people's hair – quite often that was being over-affectionate rather than aggressive. That could be difficult, very challenging even for Lucinda and I. Or he'd pull my ears …

L: He was scratching.

J: … and not let go, or grab hold of his hair, really pull at it and not let go. Sometimes we had to restrain him, sometimes he would throw himself on the floor. We would say, "Well, you are going to have to go to your room, Jim," and then he'd lie on the floor and refuse to get up. Then I'd have to manhandle him up the stairs. Obviously when you are getting older and he's getting quite big, it's challenging, something Lucinda couldn't do.

L: He quite often would bite us, bite himself … and the escorts in the taxi. We had to take his shoes off sometimes so he couldn't throw his shoes.

J: Oh, yes, he'd throw his shoes from the back of the car into the front of the car.

L: He banged his head on the window of the car so they had to put him in the middle of the taxi so that he couldn't reach.

And did you ever get any advice or help and support about how to manage all of that apart from prescribing drugs or sedatives?

L: I don't think we were ever asked, were we?

J: I don't know. I think anger-management therapy would be appropriate, really.

Did the service offer any counselling, therapy support to either or both of you?

J: Lucinda went to the doctor to get antidepressants, if that counts. She's been on them for years.

So how long ... if you don't mind my asking, how long have you been on them?

J: Decades.

When you were on antidepressants, presumably you were reviewed, did the health-care professional have any questions about why you were on them?

L: I don't know if they asked. I kind of made an excuse for having them. So it was "I've got a full-time job" and ...

And you are looking after Jim. Did they pick up on it at all?

L: No, they just prescribed more.

Did anybody ever ask you, apart from friends and family members, how are you and how are you coping?

J: People would say, "We don't know how you are coping." [laughs]

Justin and Lucinda talk about Jim's death, aged 36.

J: The scenario was this, basically. We returned from Turkey. Jim had been in respite. When you are with somebody you don't notice how much change takes place on a day-to-day basis, it's very little but over a longer period it's marked. But his condition had worsened in terms of his inability to keep food down. I was always aware of the fact that there was a danger of somebody, particularly if they were asleep, ingesting their own vomit, so that was always an issue. Clearly, we didn't know at the time when he'd been in respite that he'd had had an incident or two of vomiting. Was that right, Lucinda, when he was in respite?
L: Yeah. Four o'clock he came back, he was with us on Tuesday night and we went to the centre on Wednesday and when he came back from the centre he was very [mimics Jim's breathing], wasn't he?
J: Yeah.
L: And he wouldn't eat his tea.
J: Anyway, he got up ...
L: After his bath.
J: ... walking along the landing, clearly struggling to breathe. He wanted to go into the bathroom and he collapsed on the floor and he stopped breathing and went blue, didn't he? And I gave him mouth-to-mouth, at which point he brought up some fluid and made a slight recovery but he was still struggling breathing. And I said to Lucinda, "Phone for

an ambulance." In the past, we've got first responders and they've been really good and they would be out within ten minutes.

L: And quite often it's someone who knows Jim, isn't it?

J: Yeah, it was. Long-standing friends, actually, people who used to be in the same babysitting circles. They just don't have the people anymore in first responders ... Somebody came eventually and shortly after that the ambulance arrived and they asked, you know, the type of questions they needed to ask and we answered them as best we could and I went with him in an ambulance. I sat in the front with the driver and the other ambulance staff were in the back with him. They gave him an oxygen mask.

We got to the hospital; we were taken into intensive care, I think. It might have been, I don't think it was A&E. He was in a cubicle and was obviously in distress. They tried an oxygen mask on him but he wouldn't keep it on and I had to hold it on. Then he vomited and he basically stopped struggling, he gave up. The consultant came and said, "Clearly he's in a bad way," and he said, "We could put him on life support but if I do that he'll probably be on life support forever." He said, "Really I think that ..." He gave the impression that he'd looked up something about Robinow syndrome, but obviously, as I said, Jim didn't particularly conform to that and I knew the reason why he was struggling and what had happened. Because I said he'd probably swallowed some vomit or a lump and it's gone down to his lungs and that was why he was struggling breathing. But, you know, I explored afterwards why he couldn't do anything, like you do. And so I said to him, "Well, if that is the case, well, there's no point in prolonging his life just for the sake of it," which is a very difficult thing to say, isn't it? So he said, "Go and hold his hand," and that was it, really.

J: The issue afterwards was when we went to the registrar's office to register the death, we'd been given an envelope and taken it to the registrar without looking at it. The cause of death was Robinow syndrome and we both were taken aback because we were just shocked that was the cause of death and we didn't think it was the cause. Then I phoned the hospital and asked to speak to the consultant because I wanted to ask why he'd put that on the death certificate.

In the meantime, before I actually got to speak with him, we did a lot of research. And of course after thirty-six years there's a lot of information available on the Internet about all sorts of things. And so we discovered that one of the things that with people with Robinow syndrome was that they had restricted orifices. I mean that was one of the reasons why ... because he used to suffer with constipation, for instance; why he couldn't breathe. All those things must have been, in a way, related to Robinow syndrome but unbeknown to us, because we thought his acid reflux and his other things, his digestive problems, were something separate. So when I spoke to the consultant and he explained why he put that on there and he said, if you want to go and see if the coroner will ask for a post mortem you can do that but bear in mind that will prolong things, maybe for weeks, before you can have a funeral, et cetera, et cetera. We discussed this and said, "No, we accept that decision now and we have a greater understanding about what his condition could involve."

L: The registrar was excellent, wasn't she? She was very kind.

J: She said, if you are not happy with that, you go back to the hospital.

And that's what you did?

J: Yeah, straight back to the hospital and said we are not happy and we want to speak to the consultant. I spoke to him on the phone afterwards and he was very, very upset because you could tell that it had been … it was a difficult decision for him to make as well.

About whether it was correct to put the cause of death as Robinow syndrome?

J: Yeah … I mean, at the end of the day it doesn't make any difference, does it? We were only concerned that we thought it might reflect on anybody else who might have a child that's got Robinow syndrome, that they would get worried about things that might need not worry them at all. Because so many people with Robinow syndrome, all the other cases that we'd ever looked at, no child ever had learning difficulties. And the reason why we believe (and we didn't mention this earlier) he possibly could've had brain damage because they took some time to get him breathing when he was 4. So lack of oxygen could have caused brain damage. And there's no other documented case that we can find of anybody who had Robinow syndrome having learning difficulties.

L: Slow learners.

J: Not severe learning difficulties.

So it was only after Jim's death that you went back onto the Internet and had a look at things. Do you think that was helpful in a way, not to track it closely over the years?

J: I did try once. There was an organisation in America and I emailed them and I asked a question about whether or not any of their members of their organisation had severe learning difficulties but I never got a reply.

So, looking back, do you think it was helpful to you that you weren't aware of Jim's progressive physical decline?

J: It wouldn't have made any difference. You have to deal with those things as and when they arise, don't you?

And that last communication with that hospital consultant – that helped you?

J: He said to me, I'm here if you ever want to discuss anything with me again ... you know, this was a personal thing, he didn't have to do that professionally, he'd done his job, hadn't he? You know, at the end of the day, everybody has to come to terms with death and there's always question marks afterwards, aren't there about things, but you think, oh well, if it's not that it's the other. It's pointless really, isn't it?

After Jim died, did you have any contact with the GP surgery at all about Jim?

J: They sent a letter of condolence.

Did that feel right?

J: I thought that was quite touching, wasn't it, I thought. Lucinda, didn't you?
L: Yeah. When I went to take Jim's medication back to the pharmacy, the pharmacist came out and gave me a hug. Another nurse came past and gave me a hug and actually we went to see a doctor afterwards and we had a double meeting, didn't we? Afterwards, the consultant said he was sorry about Jim.
J: You know, we've been with that practice for well over thirty years and obviously lots of things have changed in that time. But ... some of the GPs we don't know at all, but the people we've had contact with there have always been really helpful.

Story 5: Eve

This is a story fragment about Eve who displayed symptoms of diabetes as a small child that were missed until the family moved home and registered with a new GP practice.

Eve: I was 10 … It was my mum, really, that found out … She kept taking me to the doctor, and I can remember one day in particular going out with the school and having to ask the teacher for a drink. For some bizarre reason that stays in my memory 'cause I was so, so thirsty when my sugar was high. Because I was an only child I think everyone was treating my mum as if she was a kind of neurotic mum, and they kept saying, no, there's nothing wrong, no, there's nothing wrong. And we were living in Huntingdon at the time, and then it was when we moved to London that we went … I think we went to a doctor's about something else, and he said, how long has she been diabetic? And my mum said, what do you mean, diabetic? And I was then sent straight along to the hospital.

Story 6: Finbar and Eileen

Eileen's son, Finbar, has scoliosis, which is curvature of the spine. It is usually painful and becomes more noticeable as the child grows. When serious the condition can only be treated by having a complicated operation in a specialist unit. Eileen has found the long wait stressful and has had to chivvy the NHS along to get an appointment with the spinal specialist. The support group that she joined was helpful. A physiotherapist spotted that Finbar might also have Marfan syndrome; this wasn't picked up by the other specialists.

So how old is Finbar now?

Eileen: Sixteen. He's been diagnosed with scoliosis, which is curvature of the spine, which I noticed last August when we were on holiday. He's been to see the GP and then he's been referred to the spinal specialist at XXX for fusion surgery.

When we went to the GP, she had a look at him, confirmed that, yes, she thought it was scoliosis, and then the next stage is then to refer him to the paediatric consultant at the local hospital. So we saw the GP in August and we eventually got an appointment in December to see the paediatric consultant.

Did that feel like a long wait?

E: That was a long wait and it was like a self-booking system, so there were two hospitals that we could pick from and I wanted to pick XXX hospital, and when I went onto the system there were no appointments loaded up on there, so I had to ring through and they said there weren't any appointments at the moment, they were waiting to get some appointments created and then as soon as they were they'd send me a letter through with an appointment date.

I knew it was scoliosis, I could tell from what I'd looked at online, she sort of confirmed it but she said the next stage then was to see a specialist to see what they could do then, but she did the standard test what they do, where they have to bend over to see whether, you know, they can see like a hump on their back and things like that, so yeah. But they're not the experts in it so I knew we'd have to get referred.

So we went to see the paediatric consultant in December who had a look at him, did some tests on him, his reflexes and things like that, confirmed that, yes, it was scoliosis and that he would then need to be referred to a spinal specialist and they would refer him to XXX. In the meantime he had an X-ray, and they said, yes, he's got a curve, they couldn't say how many degrees it was, they said that would be for the spinal specialist to confirm, and they said he would also have an MRI scan. So they referred him to XXX and then we had an MRI scan in December and then we got an appointment through for XXX for April this year, which I felt was quite a long wait … yeah, so it's August 2018, we then saw the consultant in December 2018, and finally got an appointment at the spinal specialist in April 2019.

Is scoliosis one of those conditions where as soon as it's been diagnosed, treatment earlier rather than later is a good idea …?

E: It depends how severe the curve is, because they say if your curve is more than 50 degrees, then it's classed as serious, and normally then you would probably have to have surgery. If it's less than 50 degrees, they can monitor it more and you can have a brace and that can be more monitored, but once it gets to over 50, they say that you would probably be better off having the surgery to correct the curve. It can be painful and obviously it's … because he's at that age like 16, it's like image, so he's twisted and … his shoulder blade sticks out on one side.

When he has clothes on, you can see his back that his shoulder blade sticks out and he has a little bit of what they call a rib hump at the back where it's pushing towards one side because the spine is curving. And you normally notice it when they're teenagers because it's when they have a big growing spurt.

The type that he's got is adolescent idiopathic scoliosis, which means that they don't know why they get it, but it's just common in teenagers, normally girls more than boys, and that they don't really know why but that's when it's noticed with a growing spurt.

The pain's got gradually worse because his curve has got gradually worse, so at the moment ... he says he's really uncomfortable after he's been sat down for quite a while because he can't rest his back against a chair properly because his back's not straight. And then also when he does sport and things, after a while it can hurt but he plays badminton and the doctors and that said you've got to just carry on as normal with everything because it's not weak or anything, your spine, it's just that it's disfigured.

So he does still carry on and they say that's the best thing, to carry on as normal and do everything that you normally can. And he went away to space school in the summer and he was doing things like scuba diving and indoor flying and he said that that did cause a few problems with his back and he was really sore. So it's limiting of things now ...

He's also been under the physiotherapist because he was having pain and they're trying to get his core muscles strong for when he has the operation, and the physiotherapist noticed that he's got very thin and quite long limbs and fingers and high arches in his feet and she wondered whether he might have some genetic problem like Marfan syndrome. So we're also linked to this, we're also going to see the genetics clinic in XXX in December to see about that and he might have to have a blood test and have some genetic testing, and if he has got something like that, then scoliosis actually is a link with Marfan syndrome, so we're not really sure yet.

For the scoliosis it's been a long delay, I think. It's the fact that having to go to the consultant and then they then have to refer you, I don't understand why the GP couldn't have referred us directly to XXX, to the spinal specialist. I'm on a forum with other people whose children have got scoliosis, so I knew that this was the process and a lot of people said it takes such a long time and it's so frustrating, because you know that they've got it, but it just takes all that time to actually get a confirmed diagnosis, and it's that in between stage.

I'd read that people say that's just the way it is and I did ring the specialist and see whether there were any earlier appointments or anything like that but that was the earliest appointment that they had on the system, so I got the appointment through in January for April.

Finbar's all right about it at the moment, I think because he's now seen the consultant and he's explained everything, and because he knows that something is going to be done. He's going to have fusion surgery on his back where they put rods in his back to straighten his spine, so it's quite major surgery.

When we first went to the specialist, they said roughly around twelve months' waiting list, so we knew it was then going to be another twelve months before he actually had the operation, so that was April, and I got an email from them this week to say that they'd looked at the list and they can probably do his operation in January/February next year [2020].

I think he was classed as a severe case, so he was on the urgent list, which is six to nine months.

So how do you feel about how the care has been organised for Finbar, so far?

E: The care is good, it's just the wait, it's just such a long wait for things like that, and to see him in pain … you just want it done as soon as possible. It feels like it's just such a long time from us knowing and seeing the GP to actually seeing somebody, and then even a further twelve months to actually get the operation. But the care has been good, it's just the slow process …

Can I ask you, because you're obviously very informed and you know how to get the system to work for you, how many times do you think you've got involved to speed things up?

E: So for the initial one with the paediatrician, I probably had to contact them about three or four times because they didn't have any appointments so I kept ringing to see whether any had been added to the list.

And do you think that as a result of that, you managed to get Finbar slotted in a bit earlier than might otherwise have happened?

E: I don't know really, because every time they just said no, there weren't any appointments and you'll get an appointment through, so they wouldn't actually give me one over the telephone, so I still had to have something sent through the mail. And then the one for the spinal surgeon came through fairly soon, I just thought, well, I'm not going to change that one, I'm just going to have to keep that, I rang up once to see whether we could get anything any sooner and she said, I'll take your details if there's any cancellation, but there wasn't any. And then it's probably now that I'm chasing more because I'm wanting to see where he is on the list … I did chase quite a few times for the results of his X-ray, so he had his X-ray in August and I didn't get an update until October, and I think I rang four times …

It's frustrating and worrying as well, because you just want everything to be sorted, and the operation to be done and then you can move on. And especially when you see your child when they're in pain.

I rang the GP because he was getting a little bit of pain and that's when they then referred him for physiotherapy.

Has the physio been helpful?

E: Yeah, very helpful, and the physiotherapist was really good because she's the one who's actually noticed the other things regarding like the genetic side of it, so it was her; nobody else had said anything about that …

Years ago when he was about 8 years old – well, no, when he was born – he had problems weight bearing, so he had to go and see the specialist in XXX when he was about 2 years old because he wouldn't weight bear, and they said he had high arches in his feet so he had some shoes made and then he could walk. And we were under the specialist for about a year and then they said, he's fine now, there's no problems, what will happen is probably when he's about a teenager he might just get some aches in his feet, so we never thought anything of it. And when he was about 8 or 9 I noticed that he couldn't straighten his fingers, they're like a little bit bent and they can't straighten them fully, so we went to see the doctor and the GP just said, everything's fine, there's not really a problem unless … she said something like, unless he wanted to be a piano player, then everything will be fine. So looking back now, there obviously was something but nobody like linked it or picked it up and it's only because he's a teenager now.

Marfan syndrome is a genetic syndrome that affects some connective tissue, and usually they're quite tall, very thin, got long fingers … their arm span, if they put their arms out, their arm span is longer than their height … so he has quite long arms. He has said people at school have commented about it and he always says my hands look funny, and he has got really long fingers, but I just thought that was his build and he's a teenager so they're growing, they are skinny and things like that. And because I knew about his feet and things but just thought, well, there's nothing, you know, everybody's said he'll be fine, but actually now … they might not be, but …

It's like a long-term condition, they say that it can affect your heart, your aorta can become enlarged or something, so you would have to have regular ECGs and things like that, so that's the bit that I'm concerned about with that side. And that obviously was only picked up with the physiotherapist, that wasn't picked up with the spinal surgeon, with the paediatrician, with the GP, nobody picked that up at all, it was the physiotherapist that pushed to get him referred. So she referred him back to the GP and the GP contacted me and said, it could be Marfan, so I will arrange for him to be tested.

The physiotherapist is really good and she's been really accommodating with appointments. And she also referred him to get some insoles with his feet as well, so the orthotist. So there's been quite a few things that have gone on with him and it's all happened at this age.

Eileen goes on to talk about how helpful it's been to be part of an online support group:

E: It's a Facebook group that I found that is a closed group for parents whose children have got scoliosis, and that has been the best information, and I do put a few posts on and get responses from people who are all in the same situation, that's the people that say, keep chasing, do this, do that, you'll be waiting twelve months, it is a slow process. So it was all people with past experience that has helped more than the actual system.

CHILD HEALTH: REFLECTIONS AND RESPONSES TO THESE STORIES

Immediate questions

1. What examples of kindness and compassion – or the opposite – particularly struck you in these stories? How did they make you feel?
2. What do these stories tell us about communicating complex information to parents? How to judge what is the right amount?
3. Why did the cause of Jim's death matter?
4. Is it important for patients and families to know "who is in charge" in a hospital setting? How is this best communicated?
5. Are healthcare professionals aware of what annoys and alarms patients and parents in a hospital setting?

Strategic questions

1. How can personalised and age-appropriate care be designed into services?
2. Why is continuity of care so important for children and their families?

3. What can be done to speed up processes of diagnosis and treatment, for example looking at Finbar's story as told by his mother Eileen?
4. What responsibilities does the NHS have to ensure a joined-up service for young people who also need support from social and educational services? How can these responsibilities be met at different levels?
5. What are the NHS's responsibilities in relation to the physical and emotional needs of parents? How can they be met?
6. How might COVID-19 have affected non-COVID care for better or worse in Dan's case? Are there longer-term implications for the design and delivery of services?

REFERENCES

Bryar, R.M., S.A. Cowley, C.M. Adams, S. Kendall and N. Mathers (2017) "Health visiting in primary care in England: a crisis waiting to happen?" *British Journal of General Practice* 67 (656): 102–103.

Colver, A., T. Rapley, J.R. Parr, H. McConachie, G. Dovey-Pearce, A. Le Couteur et al. (2019) "Facilitating the transition of young people with long-term conditions through health services from childhood to adulthood: the Transition research programme", *Programme Grants for Applied Research* 7 (4), www.journalslibrary.nihr.ac.uk/pgfar/pgfar07040# (accessed 4 January 2021).

Council for Disabled Children (2019) "It takes leaders to break down siloes: CDC's new report on integrating services for disabled children", https://councilfordisabledchildren.org.uk/help-resources/resources/it-takes-leaders-break-down-siloes-cdcs-new-report-integrating-services (accessed 4 January 2021).

King's Fund (2017) "What policies are needed to improve children's health?" 30 May, www.kingsfund.org.uk/publications/articles/big-election-questions-children-health (accessed 18 December 2020).

NHS (2019) *The NHS Long Term Plan*, Version 1.2 with corrections, August, www.longtermplan.nhs.uk/wp-content/uploads/2019/08/nhs-long-term-plan-version-1.2.pdf (accessed 3 January 2021).

Public Health England (2018) "Health profile for England 2018", research and analysis, 11 September, www.gov.uk/government/publications/health-profile-for-england-2018 (accessed 3 January 2021).

Royal College of Paediatrics and Child Health (2019) *State of Child Health in the UK* (London: RCPCH).

Smith, J., F. Cheater and H. Bekker (2015) "Parents' experiences of living with a child with a long-term condition: a rapid structured review of the literature", *Health Expect* 18 (4): 452–474.

WHO (2008) *World Health Report 2008 Primary Health Care: Now more than ever* (Geneva: WHO) https://who.int/whr/2008/en/ (accessed 29 December 2020).

MANAGING A LONG-TERM HEALTH CONDITION AS AN ADULT

INTRODUCTION

Advances in public health and medicine have done much to reduce premature death in recent decades. But we have not abolished chronic illness – whether inherited or brought on through the stresses and excesses of modern living and exacerbated by inequalities. The result is that long-term conditions have become one of the defining challenges for modern healthcare systems. In England, although it is hard to obtain exact figures, more than 15 million people are estimated to have at least one long-term condition (King's Fund, 2013) and it is becoming more common for people to have two or more conditions.

Though chronic illness increases with age, it affects all age groups and is more common – from an earlier age – among those in the most deprived areas. Patients report how disruptive and hard it is ("the treatment burden") to adhere to treatments which affect them physically, socially and emotionally, and thus how they come up with acceptable workarounds ("rational non-adherence") which can adversely affect outcomes (Demain et al., 2015).

People with long-term conditions account for a very high proportion of all health service usage. Yet those services often struggle to provide what is needed. The NHS is typically organised to deliver single episodes of care along single disease pathways. Or, as the NHS *Five Year Forward View* (NHS, 2014) put it: sometimes the health service has been prone to operating a "factory" model of care and repair. Chronic illness and multi-morbidity require different approaches. Medicines and treatments matter, but so do other factors: a collaborative approach from the professionals that is sensitive to your preferences and your experience of living with your conditions; continuity of care and the joining up of different services; being empowered and supported to manage your own condition. And above all: being seen as a whole person.

THE STORIES

These approaches and attitudes are mirrored in our Chapter 1 (Section 2, p. 4), where we offer a description of patient-centred care, in general, as:

- Understanding and valuing what matters to patients
- Seeing the whole person
- Respecting people's rights and autonomy
- Being customer focussed

There are five stories in this chapter. **Katie** has had Type 1 diabetes for around twenty-five years. **Tim** is in his 30s and has epilepsy. **Joanna** has various long-term conditions, including a rare condition. **Jasmin** has lupus and **Venetia** lives with chronic fatigue syndrome.

Story 7: Katie

Katie has had Type 1 diabetes for about twenty-five years and lives with a variety of difficult, painful and personal complications of the disease. Katie describes her ups and downs in battling to get the care she needs. The importance of continuity of care from her GP surgery is illustrated. She also talks of the impact on her mental health of living with her debilitating and gradually deteriorating condition for such a long time.

Katie: My name's Katie. I'm 50 and I've been diabetic for twenty-six years. I was admitted to hospital with very high blood sugars, just coming back early off my honeymoon. I went into a diabetic coma, basically.

And that was the first you knew?

K: Yeah.

And thinking forward to the care that you get now from the NHS, can you tell me what is the best thing about the care?

K: I'm actually seen more than I was when I was first diagnosed. Albeit that sometimes I have to push to get seen. But yes, I am seen more regularly. And the treatment out there is better. It's progressed in the twenty-five years.

I'm seen twice a year at the surgery. And a full twelve-month check, that being my feet, checking if I've had my eyes checked, and then every six months my HbA1c, whereas on the twelve-month I have a full blood check. So yeah, I am seen regularly there. This is through my GP, and then I'm also seen through the hospital, through the diabetic nurse. She sees me every four months.

And if I've had any problems, be it my eyes, my feet, I get seen quick. And when I say quick, with my feet it's within a week with the chiropodist. I am down on a six-week check, but if I've got any problems, I'm seen within the week because I've got a red flag on my records. And with my eyes as well, I just ring my optician and he's very good. I see him within the week, usually. And if there's a problem, I'm directed to the hospital if need be.

It reassures me a lot because there's a family history of amputation. And with my eyes, I've lost my licence on two occasions because I've had problems, and I know losing your licence isn't the best thing, but I know there's been a problem. And on one occasion they found out I'd had a minor stroke, so that was reassuring really, that I'd seen somebody.

When you phone the surgery, is it easy to get an appointment?

K: Usually, yes. Because again, I've got a red flag; it's like when I had the flu, I was triaged and that reassured me ... I was told that, yes, I'd got the flu, but it did progress into chest infections and different things, but because of that I was seen by a doctor, yes.

Tell me about how the nurse at the GP surgery is helpful, or not.

K: She's very good. She's actually worked with both the consultants I've seen ... She's been one of the nurses at the hospital. And then she's come out and gone into GP practice. So she knows the two consultants very well. And she also knows my community diabetic nurse. So she can liaise with them ... if I have a problem ... And she's thorough as well. I've got every faith in her, which is a good thing, because I haven't in one of the other nurses, the hospital diabetic nurse ... When I try to get hold of her she doesn't always return my messages, and I've been having a lot of problems with my blood sugars. They've changed my insulin, so obviously, my blood sugars have been up, down, and trying to get hold of her is important. Even though she's given me her email address, she's still not getting back to me quickly, because I would say within two to three days she should be getting back to me, not within a week, or even more.

At the surgery, I can usually see one of three GPs that know me. So I get the continuity. I don't have to go round and explain everything, and they know exactly what's wrong with me. All right, yes, it's got it in front of them on the screen, but they know I've been in and I've cried or … so they know exactly how I am. I just feel comfortable going and knowing that they're all really caring GPs as well. Other GPs in the surgery, yeah, they're okay, but they've known me for a long time. I mean, one of them, I've known for a long, long time and I could say she's a friend as well, and she knows the family, so it's … yeah, that's good.

Could you explain briefly how it physically affects you, your diabetes?

K: I have neuropathy in my hands. It's where the nerves die – well, I think it's what they say. So I have that in my fingers. I have it in my feet, in my toes it is really bad. And you get excruciating pain from it. I'm on medication for it but it's come to the point where it isn't working. I've had that probably about fifteen years. I've got numbness in my feet as well, and in my hands, but in my feet you have to be very careful. You've always got to have something on your feet, slippers … You can get something in your foot and not know about it and then you get infections, so it's … yeah. So that's the neuropathy.

I've got problems with my eyes. And … that was just retinopathy. I've had my eyes lasered twice, once in each eye. What else? I've got gastro-paresis … which is to do with how, when you eat, how your food goes through your tummy into the bowel, and it's where, again, the nerve endings are dying off, which causes a lot of pain, also causing problems with me going to the toilet, having my bowels open probably every five to six days. So that's another condition. I've also got problems with my bladder. Again, they've said that's to do with the nerves. So basically, a lot of it is to do with your nerves dying off.

With the bladder, I've got no control. I mean, at night I'm soaking, and that's one of the things that is really getting me down. It's one of the worst parts of it …

Is there any source of support or help for that?

K: I'm under a consultant. I'm due to start some treatment. It could work. It's a twelve-week nerve treatment again, where they put in a needle into the tibial nerve to try and stimulate the bladder. If it's going to work, it's going to work by week five. If it's not, I don't know what's going to happen, but I have got support, so … But I just wish something would wave a magic wand … Because that's the one that gets me down. I mean, well, my husband as well. Changing the bed two or three times a night … and when you're 50 you don't want that.

No, indeed. Have you been hospitalised with any of the complications as a result of your diabetes?

K: I have, yes. If I've had a chest infection I've been hospitalised. They gave me fluids and I needed antibiotics. But also, if I've had problems with my tummy with the gastroparesis, I've been hospitalised. If I've had a UTI [urinary tract infection], I've been hospitalised. Just for something simple like a UTI, you think, why are you hospitalised? But they've had to put me on antibiotics …

So how many times do you think you've been in hospital in the last twenty-six years? Or have you stopped counting, really?

K: I've stopped counting because I've had problems with my legs. I've had compartment syndromes in both my legs, which is a very rare condition. It's usually if you've had a car accident or a sports injury, but I had a spontaneous compartment syndrome in both legs and I was in hospital for nine weeks. It's when your muscle is covered in a fascia, which is like webbing on a leg of lamb … it's a very thin, but very tough sheath. What happens is you bleed within that sheath, but you've got four compartments and there's nowhere for it to go. So your leg just expands and expands, and you can lose your leg, and I was very close to losing my right leg. And I was lucky that the nurse at our local cottage hospital had worked in A&E and she said we need to get you to A&E now. So we went straight to A&E and they said they think I've got compartment syndrome, but they'll leave me for an hour. But within half an hour I was on the ceiling. The pain was excruciating and I was in surgery within the hour. They just cut the leg open, basically to … get rid of the blood. She basically saved my leg. Because if I hadn't have gone straight to hospital … So I was in hospital nine weeks for one leg and seven weeks for another, but a lot of it was because of healing.

They say the longer you are diabetic, the more you suffer from these complications. Because I've not been well with other things my blood sugars have been out of control a bit. And you do get problems because of having raised blood sugars.

I inject four times a day. And I use a blood sugar monitor, but I also use a continual blood sugar monitoring system, which isn't on the NHS. Well, it's just been brought out into the NHS. I think it was November of last year. But I've been using it probably nine months now. Initially, I was given the monitor by my diabetic nurse at the GP surgery. And she said that if I wanted to carry on using it, I'd have to pay for it, which it's about £55 every two weeks. So what I do is I use the continual monitor for two weeks and then go onto my normal glucose monitor where I have to prick my fingers. Which isn't the best because I've got very tough skin on my fingers. I can't get the blood out very good. But I can't get the continual monitor on the NHS.

And you're choosing to have two weeks on, two weeks off because you can't afford it all the time. Is that what you're saying?

K: Yeah.

What difference does the continuous glucose monitoring device make?

K: There's no finger-pricking at all, you just put the device in once and it lasts fourteen days. And it's a little sensor – smaller than a mobile phone – and you just swipe it over ... so you've got one bit in your arm and the other bit that you carry around with you. And then when you want to do your blood sugars, you just flick it on your arm and swipe it and your blood sugar's done there and then.

It also tells you if I hadn't done my blood sugars half an hour ago, it'll tell you what my blood sugars were half an hour ago. So I've got a day's worth all the time. So I can see what my blood sugars were even while I'm sleeping, which is better than having to wake yourself up because the doctor says, oh, you've got to do it during the night ...

It's made a difference that I can tell my diabetic nurse exactly what my blood sugars were. I can send her the data and she can then say, right, Katie, alter by two units or whatever, so ...

Thanks for all this. We've talked about things that have been quite helpful. What is not helpful about how the NHS system works for you?

K: When I go to see a hospital consultant, not always having my records in front of them ... more often than not, I think.

What, they don't have your records, so how do they know about you?

K: They've got basic information about me ... and I go regularly, so it's whether they haven't got them out of the filing room or wherever ... if you're not well, the last thing you want to do is sit and try and tell them what's wrong with you.

In the hospital, I've got two diabetic doctors I see. I've named one as one I would like to see all the time. I've got my ophthalmic ... I always see the same one. And the gastro, I always see the same one. But on others, it's hit and miss. And it's just going through how you've been and my ophthalmic, he knows me, so he can tell if I'm not well. And I know that it isn't always possible to see the same doctor because of illness and holidays but it's ... continuity of care's definitely important ...

I've got fibromyalgia as well. It's when you've got trigger points on your body and it's like an arthritic pain, but it's in the muscle, and you get fatigue with it. I get bad fatigue with it. I've only got to have a shower some days and I've got to go back to bed because I'm just exhausted. I've been on two pain-management courses. And they're all well and good but it isn't in my head, it's in my body. And I know that I've got pain, and it's all right saying, try to think positively, but when you're in constant pain, all day, every day, it's very hard. So, yes, seeing a pain consultant, which I am due to be seeing, I'm looking forward to. Not many people can say that, can they? Yay-hay.

On the psychological side, I have seen either the GP or the diabetic nurse at the surgery. Because of everything that I've got wrong with me, it's all medical and I get very depressed ... because if something else comes up or it's like when they told me I'd got the arthritis in my toes ... and the GP has asked if I want to be referred to talk to somebody. A few years ago I was actually sent to the psychiatric hospital to see a psychiatrist who actually dealt with health issues and depression ... He was very, very good. And I really wished I could go back, to be honest.

They tried to see if they can get me back there, they really did help. Because they understood when something happened, why I was getting depressed, and it was a vicious circle. I'd get an illness, then I'd get depressed. And then probably I'd be okay for a while, then something else would come up and it was just going round and round in circles and I'm never going to be any different. I'm not going to get better. But just having somebody to talk to is ... and the GPs just don't have time to sit and listen to you ...

I'd love to go back to work. I'd love to just say, I could do one morning, but I know that if I did that, I'd be useless the following day, and it's no quality of life. And I want to have some, so ...

The other thing – and you might not want to talk about this – but the other thing that just occurs to me is the strain and whether your husband has ever been given any support by the NHS?

K: No, he hasn't.

Has he been offered any?

K: No.

Story 8: Tim

Tim, aged 32 at the time of telling his story, has epilepsy, which was diagnosed when he was a young child. He recalls the challenges of being a schoolboy with epilepsy and the problems of stigma. He describes the difficulty of finding and keeping a good specialist and the importance of family and friends. He describes some outstanding examples of care. He talks about the difficulty of controlling his seizures, the pros and cons of support groups, and how epilepsy has influenced his identity.

Tim: I first found out about my epilepsy when I was over at a childminder's house and I was just playing games, and ended up having a seizure. Then because of that, went to the doctor's, had lots of different tests, some of the tests were for photosensitivity. At that point, I was found to be photosensitive, and I had loads and loads of seizures over time. And when it came to puberty, the seizures I had slightly changed and it wasn't so much about photosensitive seizures, they were seizures that were unpredictable. I'm that way now, most of my seizures, like, the most I have is two in a day, the least I have is one in two years, but at the moment they're like every few months. The worst part is how unpredictable they are. I get no warning whatsoever, but they seem to be happening round the mornings at the moment. But the pattern sometimes changes …

My mum didn't know what to do or say about the initial seizure at the childminder's. She had suspicions of what it could be but she didn't actually know, and my school, they were just as bad about that. At that time, I was about 6 or 7, people's information about epilepsy really wasn't very good back then, and my primary school did not know what to do about it. I had various seizures back then and the headmaster would even call my sister off of the playing field to come and help because the school knew that little about it.

It seemed like an unknown condition to most people. I'd have a seizure after doing the fun run and because I'd be so confused, like, let's say, where would your parents be, I'd say they pick me up after school because I was in a dazed condition even though if I was in a normal condition, I would have said I get picked up by childminders, and they'd walk me up and down the front of the school in my dazed condition trying to find my mum that wasn't going to be there. The whole thing, the lack of knowledge was quite substantial.

But then when we came to secondary school, the school itself still didn't seem to know that much, but some of the services that were being offered, like visits from epilepsy nurses, that helped a lot, because people seemed to understand a bit better, but it's only really been in the last five or ten years that people have started to understand it slightly better. It really does seem to have been a very slow progress because there's even the one half of the population that seems to think really dodgy things about epilepsy, like, are you cursed, and things like that. You've got a whole load of people who just either flat-out don't know, or think weird things about it, like my girlfriend's father thinks that I'm possessed by a djinn … Some really weird stuff.

I've had some very pleasant experiences with the NHS where the nurses have been amazing. I cannot fault the nurses and the emergency services. They have been the kindest, most lovely people you will ever meet. The paramedics are the best. Every single time they've come to the scene to help me, they have been really kind, really attentive and made jokes as they've helped you, and just made everything nicer. They made you feel safe and understood and cared for because they knew about your condition. I had a seizure in the park and they did the same. I've had a seizure at the front of the cinema and there I had people saying, is he dead and things like that. It makes you feel crap about yourself, and they come and they clear the area and they get you feeling better about yourself and help you to where you need to be.

And then there's the blood tests. I've had so many over the years. The ones who do the blood tests, if they are very knowledgeable of how to do it, you barely feel it. You don't even realise that the needle's in there sometimes. But then you get some of the ones who are very new, it's like a bloodbath. There was a student nurse and I felt bad for the guy … he missed the vein and then pulled it out, tried to put it back in again … and the amount of times he took to get blood … there was blood all over the floor because the guy just didn't quite know what he was doing …

I used to go to the children's hospital. I wasn't as much of a fan of the children's hospital because the queues were usually quite long and

I had a wait time that must have been, like, I think the longest wait time was about four or five hours, and that's just not on.

And one of the doctors there, Dr X ... he messed me up properly, like you can't have an investigation into him now because he's died, but the guy, he just did bad. He ended up overdosing me and I ended up coming into hospital for a week vomiting as a result of his overdose. I was a teenager at the time. Teenagers are a little bit grumpy, and because of that, he called my parents into a side room and asked them if I was on drugs because I was grumpy and he asked me if I was on drugs separately, and I'm like, you're going to be properly offended if someone's asking you if you're on drugs just because you're annoyed? I was annoyed because he'd asked me something else inappropriate and then he asked me if I'm on drugs which is going to make me more annoyed, isn't it? I'd never have drugs, I don't understand why anybody would voluntarily have drugs because my meds have made me have double vision before and they've made me sick before – I don't know why anyone would want to.

You do a test when you first go into secondary school to see whereabouts your intellect is; they placed me at a certain level and I was quite happy with that, and then they did a separate one later on because the drugs were affecting me, and I was in all the top classes, and it had affected my cognitive thinking to the level that it knocked me down to all of the lowest groups with a helper and I still had no idea what was going on in most of my classes. My mum kept on pleading, saying, please take him off the drugs, they're messing his head up, and Dr X said, no, he's okay, it's all right, and it was getting really close to my exams, it could have messed my life up, and eventually after the test that definitively proved that my head was being messed up by them, he said, okay, we can take them off. Luckily, my intellect came back again, but it meant that I had to do months of catch-up classes to get Cs and, just thinking about it, I could have got my grades so much better but it really messed up part of my life that I could have done better.

I've had a lot of unpleasant stuff like that doctor thing. But then again, I was saying about how nice the nurses are? While I was in being sick for that week, there was a specific nurse, she was nice beyond compare, and she kept me going because I've almost got a phobia of being sick – I really hate it – and the amount I was being sick that week, it really had me down, and she kept me going for that week, and I actually thanked her at the end of the week, I gave her a present because she properly helped. I mean, I have a feeling it's probably the same with a lot of people about the NHS. It costs too much and the wait times are too long because there are too many people going for it, but I don't reckon many people could complain about the nursing because they're brilliant.

I just hope that the older generation of doctors isn't like Dr X, because they seem to think that they know better than a lot of people and the nurses ... I mean, the nurse who was treating me, her and Mum both agreed on it and it's what ended up making me better in the end. He seemed to think he knew better than both of them and in the end, he deferred to what they said because of me being continually ill at that point. But the nurse knew better than him in the end. I just hope that those older generation of doctors listen to the nurses if the nurses actually are making sense. I hope they don't think they know better just because of their rank. That type of thing. I hope there's not a lot of pride that makes them think automatically they know better.

The doctors ... I think some of the older doctors are just ... I don't know if they're still with the times. Like Dr X also had my mum and sister come in for checks of random moles to see if there was any link between that and my epilepsy and I don't think that helped at all, to be honest.

Did you ever make a complaint about this doctor?

T: Strangely, we didn't. At the time, we just thought, well, that was annoying. We wished we had done it, in hindsight. But you can't really do something when someone's died, can you? But I also feel that suing the NHS is like stabbing yourself in the foot, because if you take money away from the NHS, it's taking money away from the people that treat you.

Most of the doctors I've had have really strongly varied and my epilepsy, they've all given suggestions and it hasn't helped ... my body seems to get used to my meds after a certain time. Like it helps for a bit, and then my body adapts and then I start having seizures at the same frequency again. One of the doctors at one point said I'm in about the 30 per cent of people that is hard to treat with meds and I was also told that at the moment I'm inoperable for surgery, because I've had a lot of scans for seeing if I was possible for surgery, and they said the per cent is very, very low that it would actually be a success because of the amount of knowledge they have on it. So we're not going with that; I don't want to become a vegetable or anything.

I've had so many tests. I went in and had the videotelemetry test, where you're in for a week. Hardly anybody was believing me when my mum was saying about having seizures on both sides, because it was usually whatever side it was happening on, my head would turn in the other direction and during that week I had seizures on both sides, because my head turned in both different directions and they were speculating after that point that they think that my epilepsy was in the frontal lobe somewhere between the left and right side of the brain. But in a lot of scans, they couldn't exactly tell whereabouts it was.

And one of the tests for intelligence, they decided that my intellect wasn't the thing in question, it was the processing speed. They said that sometimes it takes me longer to get to the answer but I always get the answer, which, yes, I was happy with that because that's what I was trying to explain to people that the tablets seemed to be dulling the speed of my thinking, which I already had figured that one out ... I suggest this to anybody: if you can, try and get a social group and have board and card game games days; it's helped my cognitive thinking speed quite a lot.

That's really interesting. So are you currently under the care of a consultant?

T: Well, we're trying to be because we ended up going through quite a few doctors and we got referred to Dr Y and he was quite decent. And then it got to a point where he started saying, if it ain't broke, don't fix it, but we felt like it still was broken because I was still having lots of uncontrolled seizures and we felt like he wasn't giving us any new options, so we said we're going to try and get another opinion. So we started going to him and a London doctor as well and we travelled down to see Dr Z. and we'd get different opinions from them. After a while Dr Y put me off his list and eventually it got to a point where Dr Z ended up saying, well, there's not much more we can really do here either.

We tried to get back with Dr Y but he's totally chock-a-block for ages. We would have probably stayed with the London hospital for a little bit longer but we ended up having our appointments postponed and postponed. We had three letters that were postponing my appointment and we just thought, this is stupid, we're not being seen at all.

So we're now at a point where we're seeing the person for my vagus nerve thing because I've got a VNS device [vagus nerve stimulation device inserted into the chest which can prevent seizures]. It flat-out doesn't stop my seizures but I do feel it helps my recovery time. That can't be anything but good because, working in retail, if you're not in work, you don't get paid and the amount of money I think I've probably lost over the years as a result of not being in work ... She's dealing with that and talking to me about my epilepsy, but we're trying to get referred back to the local hospital because we've run out of leads here. We don't have a doctor in the local hospital and we don't have one in London anymore. We're going through processes to get hold of a lady who is one of three specialists in XXX, so we might have another one soon …

… I've tried so many different meds that haven't worked or they have worked for a time and then haven't been effective after a while. I went for the VNS thing because I thought it's worth giving it a go, I mean, it's something we haven't tried. Dr Z then suggested a different medication, but I'd seen the side effects and I did not want to risk it because even though they were low chances, it can permanently change your personality or cause homicidal thoughts … I'm not going to do it.

My epilepsy, if I have a lack of sleep, lack of food or stress, it doesn't cause it but it has an increased chance, so I'm just trying to avoid things that will increase the chances at the moment.

I try to do things that will make it easier on me, like at work, I still do some things that are stressful but I'm not going to do things that will stress me to a level that's going to increase my likelihood of having a seizure. I know that after having a massive argument with my girlfriend, it's slightly more likely, or if I've had a massive cold, I am more likely. Sometimes around inoculation season, I know I should get an inoculation but I'm almost certain within a week of having the inoculation I will have a seizure. I know that for certain because it's happened every inoculation I've had, and I don't want to break the record of how long I've been seizure-free for now, because I'm enjoying a seizure-free patch now and I don't want to jinx it or anything.

In terms of getting help, if the seizure lasts too long or if I have two in a row, then they call the ambulance. My mum and dad have dealt with it quite a lot so they don't call an ambulance out straightaway. But my girlfriend is a little bit more jumpy about it because she hasn't dealt with quite as many and she is more inclined to call the ambulance, but she does try and wait for the time limit if she can. My friends have got a lot better at dealing with seizures: the ones I have known longer, they've had to stop the car and deal with it at the side of the road before, or just … well, some of my friends, I've got a friend who I've known for about twenty-seven years now and he's just got used to it over time, so he's okay with dealing with it now. They don't tend to immediately call the ambulance out.

When I do get taken in the ambulance to the hospital, they do some checks on me, if I've got injuries, which I usually do have, because I'm quite tall and I fall over and bite my tongue sometimes. In the past I've had one where I've fallen down and split my eyebrow and I had to have stitches. I've fallen into thorn bushes before.

I've had a lot of nasty stuff happen, so they usually deal with my injuries, check if I'm okay, if I've got a concussion or whatever's wrong with me, and after a while, if I seem to be coming back to me again, they let me out if my parents are there and my parents take me home, and I lie down on the sofa and they bring me some food and drink that I can actually have. Like they might give me a jelly or custard or something because if I've bitten my tongue, it really hurts to eat normal stuff at that time, so I'll just have some softer food until my tongue's not so sore. I'll have a large nap and try and have painkillers and things like that.

My mum and dad get a little bit teary because it upsets them every single time obviously ... I'm, like, that was a nice one, wasn't it? When we've had no seizures for a bit and they'll be, like, well, that's messed it up, hasn't it? And then we'll say we'll have to write all of this down. My mum's got a massive book, a seizure diary of every seizure I've ever had, and she's written down all of the details of what happened, when it happened and everything, because usually when I'm out for the count, my mum's the one that sees most of it and can tell the doctor better than me, so my partner and my mum are usually the ones that come with me because I can only tell the bits afterward, if I remember it, which is very rare, the bit beforehand, and it's usually the people who are around me that are able to tell the doctor most of the details.

I have to rely on my support network, You've got to get yourself a good support network, like your friends and family. If you don't, then the doctors aren't going to know all the details.

It properly scared my girlfriend when she first started going out with me. She knew I had epilepsy, I'd told her, but it's not really enough to prepare you for someone that hasn't seen a seizure before. My girl-friend's Muslim and I'm not of any religion; her mum and sister were fine with it because her mum's a teacher so she's dealt with people that have had epilepsy before, but the dad, he's quite superstitious ... my girlfriend's told me that he would think that I was possessed by a djinn. So his side of the family really would be very superstitious of it and think very strange things of it because they wouldn't believe what the medical community would tell them.

There is a lot of prejudice, to be honest. Almost every job that I've had has said things like, oh, we need more people like you, you're doing brilliantly, and things like that, and then the first seizure I have, within about a week they make an excuse and get rid of me. That's happened almost every single job I've had, including places that are supposed to be disability positive like the British Heart Foundation. But now I'm at Morrison's, they've been quite good. I even had a seizure at my induc-tion, and they said to me that it's okay, you can come in and redo the induction next week.

Is your GP involved in this at all?

T: I don't feel like my local doctor really knows very much because I think she's a maternity specialist and I've gone to her before and I've started talking about my VNS device and she had no idea what I was talking about and I actually saw her looking it up on Google … it loses all their credibility when you know more about a certain thing that your doctor does. I'm sure she knows a lot about maternity stuff but when it comes to my epilepsy, I really don't feel like she knows very much about it. Me and my mum probably know more about epilepsy than she does – it's a bit worrying.

She's more happy to give out some pills than she is to talk about it because I don't think she knows very much about it.

I did a campaign called "I am more than epilepsy" because of how people view you when you've got it, and I'm not going to mention all of the people that I interviewed. But the one I wanted to mention, out of all of the interviews, was a lady called A and her son B who had epilepsy and his was quite bad. It was making his development go backwards and he was forgetting things that he used to know.

I talked to A about various things because I don't think at the beginning she actually had a consultant, and there was a lot of stuff she did not know, and the hospital was quite far for her to get to. By the time we'd left, having interviewed her, she was really, really happy and on the verge of tears because she actually felt she had a link, because she didn't have the consultant. And I actually shared my email address with all of them, and I talked to A quite frequently about things to do with B. I shared my experiences of epilepsy and different things that I thought might help him and she was so happy about it.

When I made the whole "I am more than epilepsy" campaign, I initially set out to try and get an even balance of men and women and of lots of different faiths and cultures, and I totally found that difficult because of either different superstitions or taboos; I found out that there was a lot more Caucasian people going for it and it seemed like there were more men interested in talking about it. I was told about somebody who they ended up getting almost condemned by their family because of having epilepsy and people would keep them away from other people, saying that they're possessed, stay away from them.

But, as hidden disabilities, there's a lot of times where … with jobs, I've had people saying, can you make a cup of tea? Which is a silly thing to say to me because when I'm not having a seizure, like most of the time, yes, I can make a cup of tea, but for me to make a cup of tea when I've had a seizure or directly before or after a seizure is very dangerous.

So I avoid those type of job positions because I don't want to have a risk of maiming myself in some way. I've already got loads of scars, I've got the VNS scar, I've got a scar on my eyebrow, I've got a scar on my chest. I don't want to add to the list of scars. I'm sure most people with epilepsy have got scars because of similar things.

Around the end of primary school and throughout secondary school, I was on some meds, I had a lot of people saying things about me, not good things about me. I stuck up for myself because I'm the type of person to stick up for myself, but if you're a more mild-mannered type of person, you're more susceptible to bullying, and I do worry about people like that, because some of the meds that I had during secondary school made me slightly more angry because of it, so to stop me getting into trouble with teachers at school, they said, if you're starting to feel angry, tell the person in charge of the class and come to me and some-times I got put in the library and I was told to just sit there for a while until I calmed down a bit. But I don't really think that actually helped me in the long run: it was a way for the teachers not having to deal with it, because they didn't fully know how to deal with it. Teachers nowadays are a lot better at dealing with it; back then it wasn't really the greatest.

I'm 32 now. I think it's a slightly different generation. When I was going through school, if it wasn't a visible thing, people just didn't think it was there. The whole campaign of making unseen conditions known about, that's definitely helped quite a bit.

Sometimes because of some people feeling alone, they want to talk … But I do feel that, quite often, people at some of the meet-up groups go because epilepsy is their life. A lot of people that went to the group I was at had nothing else to talk about … it made them feel special or different in some way because it's like my epilepsy is me, I am this. That's why I made that "I am more than epilepsy" campaign. More young people, they need to feel like their condition is not defining them. Epilepsy is just something that you're going to live with, like an annoying friend that keeps bugging you every now and then. A lot of the younger generation want some people that they can probably socialise with and occasionally ask questions as a group of close friends that might share the same condition. I really wanted to start something up, like you might go bowling, but you all share the same condition so you can all help each other if you want to, swap phone numbers if you want, call up your friend that has epilepsy, ask a question, something like that, instead of just let's all complain about our conditions, because I don't think that's productive. Instead of being an agony aunt, you have a bunch of friends.

Tim, thank you so much for talking to me.

T: Not at all, it's nice to be able to talk to somebody who actually listens to your history …

Story 9: Joanna

Joanna has Ehlers-Danlos syndrome (EDS), a rare condition, and various associated complications. She has experienced high-handed doctors, a struggle to get a diagnosis, fragmentation of care and many attempts to get access to advice and treatment. She is the only carer for her grown-up son who shares the same disorder, and he also has autism, which significantly reduces her freedom to get out and socialise. Her son struggles with various health problems. They have found it difficult to get into an active dialogue with specialists who could help him and there have been delays in getting the right diagnostic tests.

Joanna: My recent experience has summarised for me how easy it is to overlook making something patient-centred … I've had a rash and it came and it went and it came and it went and eventually I showed it to my GP and then I got an opportunistic fungal rash with it. And also, there was something going on with my toenails that was a bit strange and they decided to check that for a fungal toenail infection, even though it was nothing like when I'd previously had one.

And, previously, I'd used pulsed itraconazole and that had been absolutely fine and it had cleared it up. So, they sent away my toenails, and it came back saying that they saw a fungal infection.

But the first I knew about it was that the GP had already ordered a prescription and because I am with Pharmacy to You, they had already processed it and sent it out to me by the time I realised what was going on. And, when I looked the drug up on the Internet, coffee was contra-indicated: you shouldn't have coffee or caffeine with it.

And I thought, oh no, three months of this drug, because it's not pulsed itraconazole, and coffee is one of my last pleasures in life. Because I'm a carer for my son, I don't go out, I can't meet friends for coffee or anything like that. When he was little, he was having huge meltdowns and I had to stop going out with my friends that also had small children. And so, I started buying really good high-quality coffee, and this is a really big part of my day. It is a ritual. I have a cup with breakfast, a cup mid-morning and a cup with lunch; and also, I have it with my paracetamol, so it's very important to me. And for three months to have to not do that at all, I would have liked to have talked about this first. So, we went to see my GP yesterday, I mean, when I say I'm in the middle of this, I really am in the middle of this. We had made the appointment three weeks ago for other things, for both my son and myself. We always make a double appointment for the two of us together.

And we were getting on quite well with talking about my son's difficulties and then he said, right, over to you. You've got the drugs now, you've got the prescription? And I said, well, yeah, it's about that. It didn't feel very patient-centred because you'd made this choice without discussing it with me first and it means I have to give up coffee and I'd rather go onto pulsed itraconazole because I've had it before, I know it works.

And he got quite defensive; and the whole appointment after that became very tense. And I thought about how am I going to talk to him about this, beforehand. I didn't want to blame him or be angry with him. I just wanted to say, hey, I don't think this one is the right one for me, I'd rather that one.

And, he's going ... what makes you think you can't have coffee with it? I said, well, it actually says it on the leaflet. And I got the leaflet out ... And he goes, oh, well, just don't take it with coffee, take it in the evening instead of in the morning. And I'm thinking, well, I've looked it up and it's not that, it's the metabolism of the coffee, of the caffeine that's the problem, it's not that you don't take it with it, it's that you don't take it at all.

But the whole appointment had become very tense and it was very difficult for me to put forward how I felt about it. I don't want to take this drug, I want to take a different drug, but also I want to have a really good relationship with my GP and I don't want to have this uncomfortable feeling, where I have to disagree with them almost ... I think a better response would have been, oh, I'm sorry. I hadn't really thought about that. Let's talk about it. I didn't mean to cause you upset, let's talk about your worries about this drug ...

This is a good GP. We've had problems with our previous GP at a previous surgery. We ended up leaving the surgery, along with a lot of other people. We depend on a GP to refer to secondary care and to help coordinate care because my son and I both have the connective tissue disorder, Ehlers-Danlos syndrome, the hypermobility type; and my son is more affected by it than me. He is 23 and I am in my 50s. It is really important that we have a good relationship with our GP and that we can trust them and that they can trust us. It was a two-way trust problem yesterday. Because I thought I could trust him but because I think he's got this drug wrong ... I'm thinking, but that's not what it says ... when I looked it up. I need to trust him, but can I? And, the way he said to me, well, where did you read this? made me think that maybe he doesn't trust me. But that's not the sort of signals that I've had from him before because before he's said, oh, I like people that look things up on the Internet, it makes my job easier.

This has now put our relationship possibly on a different footing, where I now have to almost renegotiate the trust between us. It's something you end up having to do on your own because you can't just make another appointment to chat to them about it because they are so busy.

I haven't decided yet whether I'm going to write an email to him to explain in more detail why I wasn't happy with it. I could try the drug and see what happens. Maybe it will be fine, but maybe it won't be. Maybe I need to try it to prove to him that you shouldn't be having coffee at the same time as you are taking this drug. I don't want to change GPs, and I know that people do that if they have a run-in with a GP, they just go to a different GP, but because of our conditions, it's best to have continuity of care.

The rest of the appointment did pick up again. It turns out I have a ganglion on one of the tendons for one of my fingers, and I'd had trigger finger problems and things like that. So, it did pick up again, he was able to do something physical, test my finger. So, we did both try to recover. So, I think it possibly might be fine. If I take this drug and then I don't have any reaction to it and I can still carry on drinking coffee, maybe he will be right and I was wrong. But I am still undecided how to do it.

At the same time, I'm thinking medicine shouldn't be this hard when we have long-term conditions like my son and I have … I've got hyperthyroid, so, there is that to keep monitoring; I've got osteoarthritis, I'm waiting for a second opinion from a rheumatologist. And then my son is in the middle of an investigation for an autonomic disorder, so I can't just not go back, or go back to see any old GP. We are sort of in the middle of things. And the acceptance that we are going to be in the middle of things for the rest of our lives because we've got long-term conditions.

I think the silos of the NHS make care very difficult sometimes. Because, with my son, I've done what they call the poor man's tilt-table test, so I've tested my son's heart rate and it goes above the recommended amount, which suggests he probably has PoTS [Postural Tachycardia Syndrome, an abnormal increase in heart rate that occurs after sitting up or standing]. So, I've been saying this for six years, but trying to get anybody to take it any more seriously than that has been very difficult.

We left the other surgery because they were refusing to refer us anywhere. I managed to get a referral to a respiratory clinic to eliminate sleep apnoea. We think his sleep is part of the problem with this severe fatigue he has, which is probably caused by the PoTS.

So, we end up with the respiratory clinic that says, no, it's not respiratory, we're going to send you to XXX to the neuroscience sleep clinic there. So, we have a day out there and they say, oh, it's not us. We think your fatigue is caused by a fatigue problem, so they send us down to YYY to the fatigue clinic, where they say, well, it's not chronic fatigue syndrome, you've got fatigue related to Ehlers-Danlos and probably an autonomic disorder. We think you ought to see cardiology.

And then finally, our new GP, the one that I want to trust, that I had trusted until recently, said, okay, I'll refer you to cardiology. And so, we were referred to cardiology, and then on to an echocardiogram at one hospital and then a tilt-table test at another hospital. And then we get the report from the tilt-table test and the expert consultant that deals with those says, I'm going to talk to the consultant that runs the tilt-table test and we'll decide what the best course is.

And, I'm thinking after all that, all those hospitals, all those different tests, we end up where I said we should have been in the first place, six years ago. But then again, we're back to them again talking about us without us. There's a couple of things in the report they got a bit wrong; and my son said, well, that's not right. But we're left with no way of being at that table.

And, it doesn't have to be a physical table, Skype or whatever, telephones we can use, but they are going to discuss what to do without us being there to talk about it with them. It feels like we're still being kept on the outside of the door while they are discussing it inside the room. And, if we're really lucky we get to listen through the door, rather than actually being part of the team to discuss what is going on and where we can move forward from it.

One of the things that they said was, because my son has pain in his feet, it is indicative of PoTS but they are unsure if maybe the pain in his feet caused his heart rate to go up. And my son, straightaway, when I read the report to him, he said, well, no, because the pain doesn't start straightaway. And so they've made an assumption that the pain started straightaway when he was tilted up, when it didn't; it didn't start for a few minutes, or several minutes.

I did email the consultant's secretary to tell her this and ask her to pass that information on. But one of the things that happens, and this has happened to me another time, is that you get these reports back from the consultant but there's no indication of whether or not you will be called in for another appointment or what you can do if you have any information. There's no email address necessarily given, except perhaps for the secretary. This is what we've found so hard. You want to discuss it further if you are anything like us.

Now, I don't know if the secretary is going to take the initiative to actually tell the consultant, either of the consultants, because there's two consultants involved. And yet, yesterday the GP said, why don't you email both consultants? find the other consultant's NHS email address, bypass the secretary and email them yourself to tell them that? So, we may well do that today.

I ended up having to make a formal complaint against a rheumatologist, which is why I'm seeking a second opinion, because I went to them with joint problems, trigger fingers and various other things; but also I wanted a diagnosis of EDS to be put in my notes, because I was having problems with physiotherapists, for instance, saying, what makes you think you've got EDS, there's nothing in your notes?

And I asked the GP to diagnose me because they can, because there's the RCGP [Royal College of General Practitioners] toolkit now. And the GPs refuse; they say, no, we haven't got time, we're not going to do that. We'll get rheumatology to do that. So, I went to rheumatology and the rheumatologist was twenty minutes late for the appointment and it was the first appointment for the day. So, I think he may have been distracted by something or there was something going on there. And I felt that he wasn't really letting me talk about what pain, for instance, and things like that.

But the letter came back from him saying, you probably have EDS but you definitely have fibromyalgia. And I'm thinking, no, I don't have fibromyalgia; I don't meet the criteria. And so I rang the secretary to say this and say, I dispute the fibromyalgia, but, oh, it said he was waiting for the blood test results and the X-rays. And I said, well, you're going to have a long time to wait for the blood test results, he didn't request any. And she was, oh, that's why we haven't got them back yet.

And, at the appointment he had actually said, oh, you've done all the blood tests you need at your GP, we don't need any more. We just need the X-rays. So, then the second letter comes back saying, thanks for pointing out that you haven't had the blood tests; the X-rays look fine, and didn't mention the fibromyalgia, so I thought, oh, he's dropped that one.

And then the third letter comes saying, osteoarthritis; probably EDS, definitely … and widespread chronic pain of the fibromyalgia type and that was it, there was nothing to say, to bring me in for another appointment. So there was no opportunity to discuss it. As far as I was concerned, I'd already pointed out to the secretary, which was my only contact with the consultant, that I disagreed with the fibromyalgia.

So, I rang PALS [Patient Advice and Liaison Service], the GP said, yeah, this isn't right. I also did a subject access request to get my X-rays because something didn't feel right about it and the foot X-ray actually said in the report, we need to see more X-rays because there's a shadow on there. There was a luminosity that wasn't there last time. And that was buried in the report and the rheumatologist didn't mention it.

So the GP said, go onto PALS and PALS said, well, we can ask him to reverse the diagnosis, but it might be best if you make a formal complaint at the same time if you're going to do it. So I ended up having to make a formal complaint. And how the formal complaints work, they don't talk to you, they talk to the people at PALS and PALS talk to me.

Do I get the impression you didn't really want to make a formal complaint but this is the process you have to go through?

J: Well, I thought that there was no other process to go through to get this sorted out. And he said, in his response back, I was surprised to get a formal complaint out of the blue. And I'm thinking, well, it was only out of the blue because you didn't invite me back for another appointment. I'd already expressed a disagreement with the diagnosis with your secretary. It's not my fault that she didn't pass that on to you. And he left it with, I could reverse the diagnosis but I think you should have a second opinion.

And I went back to PALS and said, would you just get them to reverse the diagnosis; so, it's taken out of my notes and I can't be bothered to go for a second opinion, this is getting ridiculous. I said, forget it. And they said, no, no, no, reading between the lines, he thinks he might have missed something. You need that second opinion.

But, in the meantime I'd been to see a physiotherapist on the advice of my GP, and she had said she just assumed everything was fibromyalgia and there was nothing wrong with me and nothing wrong with my hands. And when I asked her to look at the X-ray, she said, oh, there won't be any osteocytes on your hands. There's no bony growth because you're not hypermobile but you've got good range of movement.

And when I made her look at the X-rays she said, oh, it is an osteocytes, so, because he'd put down fibromyalgia I got poorer-quality treatment from the physiotherapist that just assumed it was all fibromyalgia and psychological rather than, actually there was osteocytes in my hand. There is a reason why my fingers look swollen; because there's lots of bony growths on them.

So, it would have been nice if, somewhere along the way, I didn't have to go through a formal complaint but there was just … have we got this wrong? Come on in and we'll talk about it again.

You are, by the sounds of it, a highly educated, motivated, knowledgeable and proactive person and if you can't make the system work for you, how is somebody who doesn't have those advantages going to make the system work?

J: One of the GPs that I've chosen not to see actually has a mug on his top shelf that says, don't confuse my seven years at med school with your Google search. Which, actually, intelligent people find very offensive. Because, don't confuse your twenty-minute lecture at medical school on my condition with my fifty-seven years of living with it.

I'm on the fringes of support groups. I don't go all-in for going to all the support group meetings, but I belong to some online support groups and I run a support group – I have done for many years – for families who home educate children who have special needs and disabilities. And a lot of them, their children have very rare conditions. There seems to be two different kinds of people that come up against these problems in the NHS. Either they become like me and they advocate for their family or their children or whoever it is, or themselves, and they get very frustrated but they keep pushing along and try to make things better.

Another sort of family are the ones that give up on the NHS and they go to alternative things, and that can get them into a lot of trouble. They end up with a quack or they end up spending a lot of money on things that don't work, or they go for scary alternative things: there is this thing of bleach for autism, and that's very difficult to watch people be forced out of the NHS because nobody in the NHS has listened to them and they haven't been able to navigate around the NHS to get the services they need.

And then there's the others that just give up. And I think my son is like that. He said, Mum, I think I just want to give up. He's got problems with his eyes; he's got dry-eye disease now. And he said, I can't be bothered anymore. The drops that worked for him we can't get anymore: they are not on the list. He's 23 but he's got autism as well and he's just like, Mum, you deal with it if you can but I just don't want to deal with it anymore. I can't do it.

Those are the people that the NHS never see again and I get the feeling that GPs and nurse practitioners and sometimes the consultants go, well, that must have gone well because I saw them and I said, well, you've probably got this and now they've gone away, so they must be fine about it. And what they don't see is the patients that talk together about how awful and how difficult the NHS is and how to navigate through it, and how to get something out of it.

I think one of the problems with a rare condition is that collectively they are very common. They start looking on the Internet and they go, wow, I think this is it. This explains everything. So, they go in and they say this to their GP and their GP says, oh no, you can't possibly have that, that's a rare condition. And I've actually had a GP say to me, but the rate of Ehlers-Danlos is 1 in 5,000 and we only have 4,000 patients at our GP surgery, therefore we can't have anybody with EDS, it's unlikely. And you think, wow, that person doesn't understand statistics and numbers.

Then there's a paper that came out recently that was done in Wales, and they found the prevalence of EDS was 1 in 500. How can it be 1 in 500 and yet the GPs are telling patients, it's very rare? And I got to thinking, maybe the GPs, they are not talking to each other and so they think, I'm really unlucky, I've got a patient that has EDS, not realising that every other GP is saying, oh gosh, I'm really unlucky I've got a patient with EDS. This idea that it's rare so you can't have it, means that the patient has to work even harder and then you start to question yourself, you start to say, well, maybe I don't have it? Maybe it is all in my mind? Maybe it is a psychological thing?

And that can be very dangerous for patients too because there is a high rate of depression found in patients with EDS and it's years of not being believed by the system that they have this condition, which was thought to be rare but actually isn't as rare as they thought it was.

We go on to talk about Joanna's son.

J: One of the things that is supposed to happen is these special, learning disability appointments that everybody with a learning disability who is registered with their GP is supposed to have a check-up every year. And they've now added autism into this as well. Most parents will say, really, are we supposed to have these appointments for the kids every year? We haven't had one. And it does seem to be a missed opportunity to have the nurse from the GP surgery sit down with the patient and their carer or parent to say, okay, so, what's going on? Can we coordinate this? Or, what are we missing here? What can we do? Who can we see that will help? For instance, with my son, if we'd had a nurse advocate saying to the GP, the tilt-table test that the mum has done, it looks like we should be going straight to cardiology. It would have saved time and money if we'd gone straight there.

In fact, they did lend us a blood-pressure cuff, and I used it to do his heart rate. And, when I gave it back to the nursing assistant at the surgery that organised it, I said, so what you are looking for here? She says, yes, I add it all up and then average it out. And I said, no, we're looking for peaks; we're looking for the outliers not the average.

And so, when she handed it to the GP and I saw it later in my son's notes, when we got his full notes access, she had averaged it out and given it to the GP as an average, which is completely not what should have been going on. And if a senior nurse, somebody who actually knows about things, had been able to sit down with us … it doesn't have to be a GP because I know they're really busy. But somebody to sit down and go through everything and get all the details and all the blood tests together, and then present it to the GP and the GP can say, okay, we know it's reliable, because we don't want to trust these parents. Because that's what it feels like, it's the parent and nobody trusts you; so, it's coming via the nurse. And then they can look at it and say, okay, yeah, let's … let's see what the most appropriate thing to do is. But it seems to be that coordination is just completely missing.

Yes, and some of the other things you were saying were making me think about care planning and the conversations that go into that, and the need for somebody with sufficient clout to advocate on behalf of the family, particularly if relationships have become rather frosty or fraught. And that would be especially useful for families that don't have the education and confidence to be able to battle the system and they might just crawl away as you were saying earlier.

J: I used to be chair of the patient participation group [PPG] at my last surgery till it was taken over; and my last act just before I left, at the last AGM we had about twenty to thirty patients in the room, plus a GP and the practice manager and assistant practice manager, and I said, what do you want to see the surgery doing over the next year? A few older patients said, well, we've got these care plans but the doctors don't seem to know about them anymore.

And so, we turned to the staff, and the assistant practice manager said, I've heard there was a pilot for these care plans a couple of years ago.

And three patients said straightaway, yes, that was really great because we were given a card, so we knew who to contact when something went wrong. The surgery would say, yes, you can have an appointment straightaway.

And the GP said, would you like to do that again, and they all said, yes, we'd like to have this care plan so that we know where we are and where you are. And I was speaking to one of these people several months later, after I'd left the surgery, and I said, so have they followed up with it. And she said, no, they didn't follow up with it.

I felt really awful that I'd left the surgery and I'd left the PPG because I wasn't able to go back and say, at the AGM you agreed that you would look into doing these care plans again. But it seems to be, in the NHS there's lots of little pilot studies and lots of little trials and, oh yeah, that really works. And the patients go, yeah, this is great, this is what we want, but there's no incentive to keep it going, or the staff change and it just disappears.

It feels that the NHS is fire-fighting so much and that they've become entrenched, everything is awful, what are we going to do? Without realising that if you just sat down and talked to the patient sometimes things would be easier, cheaper and happier. It feels like everything around you in the NHS is trying to stop you accessing services, so you are constantly fighting against that, rather than sitting down and saying, okay, so what's the best service for you? What is the best place to refer you to? Like this RCGP toolkit for GPs to diagnose Ehlers-Danlos, there's no need for the patients to actually go to a rheumatologist who probably has no interest or no experience in EDS if a GP can do it.

The conversation then turned to physical therapies for EDS.

J: Because it's a connective tissue disorder, it's something you've got for life and the physiotherapy has to be something that is done for life. And you may have some joints that act up, you may have other things that happen.

You can't be restricted to six weeks and you are discharged, or what happens now is just one appointment and you are discharged. The same happened with podiatry. We had a head of podiatry who had done a PhD and I actually read his dissertation and it was fascinating because I thought, this guy gets it. He said, we have to get away from this acute medical model of there is one thing wrong and it will be fixed and then you won't see us anymore, because that's not what's happening.

We recently had a most ludicrous situation. He has bespoke insoles made by the podiatrist but he also has boots supplied by the orthotics department. And the stitching had come apart on the boots so I rang up to see if we could get them repaired, because they are NHS property and so on. And they said, no, because it's been more than six months since you've seen the orthotics department so you have to get another referral from your GP.

So, I went to the GP and the GP says, I can't refer because there is no referral pathway in our system to refer straight to orthotics. You will have to go through podiatry, and I said, well, ironically, we are asking to see podiatry again as well, but this is ridiculous because this is NHS property. It is defective. The stitching on the boots had come undone.

If there was a cobbler on every doorstep, I could get them fixed myself but then I would be told off for interfering with NHS property.

So, they let us bring the boots in anyway, without waiting for the referral from podiatry, which is a good thing because we still haven't seen the podiatrist. Luckily, we kept my son's old pair of boots but they are not as comfortable and they don't support his ankles properly. It was about eight weeks before the boots came back. So the whole thing was a complete palaver, going round and round in circles because the system is made for the system not for the patient.

I've often said that some aspects of the NHS should be run by Ocado, because it is actually a logistics company. My groceries arrive; my order comes every week. It always comes within a time slot. I never have to wait for it, unless there's been like something, a disaster on the motorway or something like that. If they can do all that, maybe they could arrange some of the administration side of the NHS as well. It seems a bit odd that there is this idea that the NHS is too big somehow. And maybe it is, and maybe that's where things should be done more locally.

Story 10: Jasmin

It took Jasmin four years to get a diagnosis of lupus, during which time she suffered stomach and joint pains, extreme tiredness, insomnia and a recurring skin condition. During this time she also gave birth to two children. In the end a private doctor got to the bottom of what was going on. It has been a battle to get the treatment that she needs.

Jasmin: My lupus symptoms weren't taken seriously. It took about four years to get diagnosed. And by then I was in a really bad way, I felt like my whole system was shutting down and I was having problems one after another, and I wasn't quite sure what was going on but I knew for sure there was something wrong.

I used to have pain in my upper stomach, bloating, nausea, a lack of appetite, I lost weight and I used to get cramps and I couldn't sleep very well and I was really, really tired. And I used to have itchy skin which would come on my cheek and my face and I used to get it under my armpits and my forehead.

So I had lots of symptoms ... my body was all over the place, so I went to the doctor, but nothing much was done. Then the pain continued and one day it was unbearable, so I called NHS Direct. I was advised to go to the A&E, which, when I did, the tests said I had H pylori bacteria infection.

It's an infection in the stomach but I had suffered for a while before I could find that out. Then I got the treatment but shortly after that I continued getting the pains in the stomach, because sometimes it can come back, depending on maybe how long you've had it for. So, I decided to change my diet and I went gluten-free. I really changed a lot of different things just to see what was happening. Then after, I got diagnosed with irritable bowel syndrome [IBS] and hiatus hernia, but this is before they found out about the lupus. My body was just shutting down with one thing after another but the actual illness that I had, nobody could work out.

Later I got pregnant with my first son, about thirteen years ago. From the beginning of the pregnancy my lower back, the coccyx and the upper back was really bad and I was really, really tired, it was just unbearable. And my skin was very itchy and sensitive, especially on my face and I couldn't work out why and it used to swell up. So, I went to the doctor and he suggested maybe the creams I was using, or that is expected when you're pregnant to be very tired.

I took some time off work but I'd never felt like this before, it was really weird. Even walking, I felt like I was falling down into a hole … like when you feel like you've got no energy in your eyes.

I was so weak and I lost quite a lot of weight but my baby was growing normally because every time I went to check, everything was fine with the baby. So, I was lucky really because sometimes if you've got lupus you could lose the baby.

I'd never even heard of the word lupus before, so I never knew what was wrong. I think giving the doctor all the symptoms I was getting, maybe he could have put one and one together, but obviously he didn't and I didn't know. And sometimes you're just thinking, maybe am I making it up, am I crazy or what's going on? Can someone find out what's wrong with me?

After the pregnancy, I had the baby, the symptoms were still bad, so I had to have an epidural injection after the baby was born … I had to go and see an osteopath. I was doing it privately, for my back, nearly every other week … I've seen so many people … I went to a chiropractor, a physio, a cranial osteopath … I used to see them a lot … And one of the ladies who I was seeing said this is not normal, it's not right. There's something really not right with you because I see you one week and we treat you, within three or four days you're better and then you're back again.

I went back to the GP and he said maybe I need to take some time, and try to take some more rest, and painkillers. I was still suffering. He gave me different creams to try at home, maybe just to see … One time he said, maybe it's just a couple of spots and maybe it's not that bad. But I'd say to him, this is not just spots, they're really itchy, they're hurting and I feel it's swelling up.

So, I decided to go private because it was really affecting my sleep and, having a new-born baby as well, I found it really, really difficult. I told my husband, it'll be something which is going to kill me but it'd be really good to know what's going to kill me, because I didn't feel right. I used to go the baby group and I thought, I'm talking to the rest of the mums, they don't feel the same I'm feeling, so there's something really wrong with me. Sometimes I couldn't even carry the baby.

We've got private medical insurance, so I told my husband, I think we need to go and check somewhere else because I don't feel right. It was awful. Reflecting back, I felt like I wasn't listened to when I reported all my pain. So I went to a private doctor in London.

He was a dermatologist. Because I was seeing a chiropractor for my back I thought maybe if I see someone for my face, it could be sorted. Sometimes I would get big spots and they had a bit of pus, on my armpits, pubic area and on my face.

The private doctor was very good. He sent me for tests on my back, and they tested a lot of things. He was checking on where I worked, the environment I live in. I went to see him more after the summer because it was so bad. Sometimes because no one can seem to find out what's wrong with you, you just learn to just live and cope with it.

I got pregnant with my second son and the pregnancy again was really bad because my back was in a really bad way. And sometimes I would sit down and I'd have someone lift me up because when I sat down my pelvis softened. I couldn't lift myself up … sometimes people get that when you're pregnant. I was just over-exhausted. And you can't explain to someone how tired you are. And because I've always been a person who looks okay on the outside, sometimes you get ignored or people don't take you seriously.

The private doctor I was going to see was very helpful. One time I was really sore and he said, this is not normal. He took some photos and he said, I need to show this to my superior because I can't work out what's wrong.

He gave me some steroid injections to bring the swelling down and I got a bit better. He said, hmm, that's interesting. The next time I went in, he gave me another steroid injection and he said, if it's reacting to the steroid injection maybe there's something that we need to check. He asked: do your nails grow? My nails used to really grow and they stopped growing, my hair started falling out but then people say, oh well, you have babies, your hair doesn't grow as well as it used to, that's all it is. The doctor said, we need to take a biopsy ... They cut one of the spots on my face and one on my armpit and that showed I've got lupus.

I really don't know how I coped. But my husband was very supportive and I was having to go private for everything, and I had to go all the way to London every time. Honestly, trust me, if I didn't have private insurance, I would not be here today and I'm not joking. Because lupus is very serious.

Now that you've got your diagnosis, is it a condition that you can manage reasonably successfully?

J: Yes, you can with the right medication, but when they put me on the medication, because my stomach was so sensitive, and I was so malnourished, I used to get cramps. That medication, it's called hydroxychloroquine, was too strong for me and my body couldn't handle it.

The doctor had to send me to another stomach specialist, where he had to clear my gut and give me a probiotic. And I had to cover up, I can't be in the sun. He wrote to my doctor and told him, this is her condition. And I went back to the GP and I said, you see, I had something really wrong with me but you didn't believe me.

And what did your GP say?

J: I wanted to change the GP, but in the end, I just thought, actually now he knows, let's see. Since then I feel like I've been treated differently.

Sometimes I wonder what would've happened if I didn't seek private medical help. And I wonder whether gender and the different healthcare experiences of men and women had a part to play with my late diagnosis. I don't know, it's really hard to tell. I think maybe it was because of my gender, my race, my ethnicity, I don't know. You're asking yourself, why? I've gone so many times to see him ... Maybe it's because I'm young, was really hard to tell. I feel like it shouldn't have taken four years to be diagnosed with lupus. And I know lupus is a condition where sometimes it's difficult because you get so many symptoms. Maybe the doctors need to be a bit more educated and understanding about lupus, so that other people don't have to suffer as I have. I think what you can expect is that they're really keen to try and help you work out what it is.

That's how I felt with the dermatologist in London. He did everything he could, honestly.

Jasmin then went on to talk about an infection in her sinuses that went undetected, causing her to have unnecessary dental treatment:

J: At the same time with the lupus, I had problems with my sinuses. I'm really allergic. My eyes would just go watery, my nose would get blocked.

And I used to struggle more on my left-hand side, so everything on my left was so bad, from the head, from where the sinuses are on the top of the head, on the shoulder, the neck, the lower back and around my hips. And sometimes it'd be so bad, I'm not walking properly, it would start affecting my knees. So, I went to see the doctor and said, there's something really wrong with my sinuses. But for me I didn't think my sinuses was that bad, I just used to think it's in the summer. And sometimes it will affect my teeth. I used to think it's a toothache because it's like at the top of your jaw line as well. So, I went to the dentist and I just said, my teeth are really hurting so he said, let's do a root canal because it looks like you need a root canal. So, I had a root canal done and it was still really hurting. And it's expensive to have a root canal done.

Five months later it was still really hurting and I said, I don't get it, it's still hurting. And I said, it's so bad, just take the tooth out.

I had the tooth out. I was still getting the pain and I went back and I said, you know what, there's something really wrong. And he said, I need to send you to have a CT scan, it may be the sinuses, but to me it sounds like toothache. So, he put me on the waiting list. He had a look and he said, the waiting list for the sinuses at the NHS is long. I said, okay, I'll use my BUPA to go private. They saw me within five days. When the CT scan result came in, they called me and they said, emergency, you need to come and you need to have an operation.

The whole of my left side was a shadow, so they called me for an emergency operation. I used to spit yellow stuff when I brushed my teeth. And that comes of infection but because it never came out through my nose, it was just like draining into my gut, so in a way that's why I continued having problems with my stomach because all that bad stuff was draining into my gut.

The consultant removed so much, he said he'd not seen anything like it and he said, how have you lived like this? I don't get it. How have you lived like this? I said, I've been complaining but … I've had the teeth out, I've done this, I've done that, but I didn't know what was going on with me but I knew my left-hand side has not been functioning properly. And since the operation my lupus was a bit better, honestly. Because I think on top of the lupus, having all that draining into your gut every single day …

And did anybody at any point say that the two things might be related in some way, the lupus and the sinus?

J: Yes, the doctor for the sinuses said that maybe compromised my immune system. Lupus is when the body starts attacking itself, so because you're having all this bad stuff draining into your gut that the body didn't know what to do with itself, it started attacking itself ... And if you've got a family history of thyroid or arthritis it's more likely because lupus is like an autoimmune illness.

I thought, now they know what's wrong with me maybe I can have an NHS identity. I see a dermatologist, she's ever so lovely, and I see her every couple of months, where they test my blood to make sure everything is okay.

And because as well, the tablets that I take for the lupus can make you blind, I have to have regular eye tests ... I felt like one thing that has been really good in my body are my eyes. I go to a lupus group now and a couple of people have lost their eyesight, so I just keep hoping my eyes will be okay. And so far, so good.

Has the lupus group been helpful?

J: Yes, because, at the beginning, I never knew about lupus. I Googled it and, oh, my God, I'm dying. I just needed someone to talk to, someone who'd gone through ... And I didn't even know any other people ... Sometimes I find it a bit difficult because it reminds you of a difficult time. So sometimes it's good and sometimes it's not, because it depends on how I'm feeling, because I'm a very positive person.

When it comes to helping you learn to live with lupus and to manage the condition, who's been the most help to you?

J: I think my husband, and I would say that the dermatologist in London. And I'm really happy with the dermatologist I see now; yeah, she's really good, although, some things she can't control.

Story 11: Venetia

Venetia lives with chronic fatigue syndrome. She describes a lack of support for the condition, particularly from her GP. There is no local specialist clinical service and instead she researches online for information.

Venetia: I suppose it was just over three years ago now, it was over a summer. I remember I seemed to have two or three bouts of flu in a row and I was sleeping all the time, I just didn't seem to be able to recover. I went on a walking holiday in September and I was sleeping an awful lot and there was an 88-year-old who was also on the walking holiday and I was struggling to keep pace with her. On that holiday one of the other ladies took me aside and told me her story about how she'd had CFS [chronic fatigue syndrome] and how it had really compromised her life and she'd been, for a number of years, basically housebound. I'm thinking, gosh, this poor lady, that would be awful, I wonder why she's telling me about this ... I came home and I went to the doctor's, but it was probably about five months before I got a diagnosis of CFS officially.

The first year was awful, particularly before I got a diagnosis and I didn't know what I was doing. I couldn't be ill because I wasn't allowed to be yet until I had the certificate. So you're trying to fight it and you're trying to go full steam ahead and it's just like slamming yourself into a concrete wall over and over again.

So that didn't work too well. Eventually, once I started understanding a bit more about pacing and what they recommend, then things improve and I went part-time at work and that helped massively. You get used to doing a lot less. Antidepressants made a huge difference as well, because if you're saying no to everything and doing a lot less, that can be a bit depressing, so the last two years have been much better. Although I've come off the antidepressants more recently, in September, and that's been shaky. Then my latest great hope is ... I've got an appointment with an osteopath who reckons he can cure CFS. So that's worth throwing about £1,000 at. I'm thinking, if that works then great, and if that doesn't work I'm going to go back on the antidepressants and keep on my nice little slow steady even keel.

Let's talk now about what happened when you first went to the GP.

V: The first time they say, well, it's just flu, and you say, no, no, no, this has been three months now, I wouldn't have come to the doctor with flu. They say, yeah, it's probably flu. So, after you get over that hurdle ... the first time that somebody told me about CFS were the doctors there. It's something that's haunted my entire illness. I should say, with CFS, a lot of the times when you're talking to the doctors, it's really hard because your brain doesn't work, your memory's shot, you can't think logically. I remember he said, I think you've got chronic fatigue syndrome and he explained that there wasn't a cure and then the words that he used were, you just have to accept that whatever it was you wanted to achieve in your life, you're not going to be able to. That's okay, because you don't really want to achieve these things anyway. It's just society telling you that. If you really think about it, you don't really want these things. But he never at any point stopped to ask me what it was that I wanted to achieve in my life. So I promptly burst into tears like an ordinary human being and he said, I don't understand why you're getting upset. I don't understand why anyone gets upset when I tell them about this. If I tell somebody that they've got a broken leg, and they can't run a marathon, well, they don't argue with me, so why is it different for chronic fatigue? When you're feeling low, those are the words that are going through your head and they just recycle. I can see what he's saying, there is some truth in what he's saying, but it's not what you first tell somebody that they've got CFS.

I remember going to see the consultant [specialising in CFS] and I had my little list because I knew my brain wasn't working so I'd written down all my symptoms on my phone. I was all ready and I prepped and I went in. I sat down and I got out my phone and I started, … and he said, no, hang on a second, and he brought out his list and he gave me the chronic fatigue checklist and he said, tick all the symptoms that you've got. It was a big list. It was a real relief because I went down the list and there was just a few that I didn't have. So you get a sense of I'm not a fraud, I'm not making this up, look I match, I'm official.

How did you feel when he produced his list and didn't let you use your list?

V: I wasn't too upset about it at that point. It was only actually much later when my brain kicked in and I suddenly thought, hang on, I had things on my list that weren't on his list and they never got talked about. Because as soon as the checklist was done, he said, yeah, you've got CFS, out you go. That was my entire experience of anyone who is supposedly an expert in CFS, at that level. There's been no follow-up from that whatsoever. They put you then through into the chronic fatigue treatment programme which is CBT [cognitive behaviour therapy] and physio.

You have graded exercise therapy which takes place in parallel to the CBT … The eight-week course on managing CFS was fabulous. I couldn't rate them highly enough … you learn your pacing and they do diaries and all that stuff. That was really, really good. Then the next course that they put you on after that was advanced CBT and that was great as well, because you learn how to not waste energy on thoughts … and then you're considered to be an expert in CFS and you fall off the end of the conveyor belt.

So have you not been back to a doctor since?

V: I've been to my GP again.

Right, but you never saw a consultant again?

V: No.

You've never seen a specialist again?

V: No.

So do you feel that that's a gap?

V: Yes, because an awful lot of people that you talk to with CFS, they struggle for years and then all of a sudden they find out, oh, I've actually got this other thing. With CFS, they don't know what causes it, so my suspicion is that there's not one thing that's CFS, it's multiple things. Now, probably several of those are already known about, but the more unusual, it's harder to get a diagnosis for them. I've no idea what tests my doctor did, because diagnosis for CFS is a diagnosis by exclusion. I was sent for umpteen blood tests but I've got no idea what those blood tests were for or the results.

I know one was for Vitamin D because the doctor came back and said your Vitamin D's terribly low and they put me on a really high dose. Then I rang the surgery and asked to have it retested as I'd been on this high dose for a while and I got another test, I saw a different doctor. And they said, woah, your Vitamin D is off the scale, you've got way too much Vitamin D, and they looked at my original results and said, that's a perfectly normal Vitamin D result ... I don't have an awful lot of faith, to be honest. The same thing happened with my thyroid actually.

I'm not sure what else I expect them to do. But there's no follow-up ... with my GP or with anybody ... They did say that there would be follow-up things, but then the final course [on mindfulness] I actually dropped out halfway through because it was driving me mental. I tried so hard to stay on the course because I didn't want to piss them off and ... mark my card for being ... a difficult customer, patient, whatever you are. But I just couldn't cope with it anymore.

What's been a highlight or a good thing that's happened in terms of finding your way and navigating the maze?

V: Occupational health [service organised by employer, not NHS] ... It was the first time I felt that the world wasn't falling apart ... it was before

I'd got my proper diagnosis and so it was in between being told that my life was over, and my getting my actual diagnosis from the consultant. I was still bobbling along trying to do full-time work. I felt like I couldn't tell anybody that I was ill because it wasn't official yet. It got to the point I couldn't cope anymore, so I made an appointment with the occupational health department here. I went in and I felt like such a fraud and he just sat me down, he said, we're going to wrap you in cotton wool. It doesn't matter about your diagnosis; until we know otherwise, this is what you've got and we need to take care of you and make sure that we're doing everything we can to support you. It was just amazing, it was the first time anybody had, outside of my family, really been caring about it.

Have there been any other examples of people being caring, outside your family?

V: The psychologist was very good and caring. Eventually I left my GP when he told me that I needed to stop trying to get better because this is obviously what God wants for me. Yeah. So I walked out of that appointment, round the corner, into the next doctor's down the street and said, can I sign up with you, please. The first doctor I saw at the new place, he was a locum and he came across to me as really caring. The difference is that he started off asking: how is this impacting your life? None of the other doctors had asked about that. They'd not asked how I was managing at home, at work or anything like that. He said, I don't know all that much about CFS: you tell me what your experience is. It was just really nice to have someone start from that perspective. Unfortunately that doctor's surgery is closed and I'm now back with my original doctors because they'd put us all back in there. So I'm back with the ones who don't actually want me to get better.

So, given the fact that there isn't a cure for CFS, what is important to you about how the system supports you, or signposts?

V: You start looking online; you look at what's available elsewhere. I was reading about a book that's written by several people who work at XXX; they have a CFS clinic there and they've got all these leaflets and they put them into a book and I just bought this book and I thought, oh, they've got lots of really useful leaflets. You think: why is that not more widespread? Why is the good practice … I know there's a famous clinic for CFS in London … but if you're not in one of those areas then you seem to have absolutely no access to it.

I've tried to get involved in research studies because mum's got Parkinson's and she's found that being involved in the research studies is actually the best way to get ... I keep looking online and I haven't found anything. Maybe I'm just looking in the wrong place again; I don't know where to look, really. My doctors have a thing on the website saying, we're a research active practice, our patients are involved ... but ... there's no "click here" to find out more or sign up or whatever. So I went into the practice and I said, I'd like to put my name down for anything on the CFS front if there's anything going. I remember the receptionist looking at me, just like I'm coming from Mars. Nobody had ever asked this before ... I said, it's on your website. So she went off and got the manager and they came back and said, yes, we've put your name on a list and I thought: is that a list of one ...?

After the first meeting with the doctor, I wasn't in a fit state really to ask questions, so I went back and I talked to another doctor and I said, I'd like some more information. He said, oh well, I don't really know, but there's plenty of information online, you can just Google it. I thought, really, okay. So I went home and I Googled it and that was a horrendous experience. I know a lot about it now, I know which sites are better ones, more optimistic ones, for me to look at, but there's a lot of militantism on the Internet with CFS.

I remember one of the first things I read was somebody saying, if you recover from CFS then you never had it in the first place. I thought, well, okay then, I don't want CFS, I'll have whatever the mystery thing is you can recover from, that will be fine. I think that was to do with the ME Society. There's a forum I go on called the Patient Forum, which is basically just other patients ... I remember I put a link to some scientific journal and that got held up for three days while obviously somebody checked that it was bona fide.

What difference would really good signposting, navigating and support have made, or would make in the future?

V: I think the most important bits could have been at the beginning, because you really don't know what's going on. Also for a lot of people that's when your symptoms are at their worst because you're not managing them at all. So your brain doesn't work, you really need neon flashing signposting. The occupational health guy that I saw gave me the booklet with official NHS NICE guidelines. It was a really clear guide: okay, we don't know what causes it, but these are the symptoms, this is what you need to do, there's boom and bust cycles, this is your graded exercise therapy. It was about five pages, but just having that ...

that's what the doctor should have given me, instead of telling me to Google it ...

How come you've ended up going to see an osteopath?

V: My uncle sent me a link to a Sky News article ... you get a lot of advice from a lot of quarters and most of it's really ... well, if you did it all, then you wouldn't have any energy for anything else, or any money because a lot of it involves buying nutri blenders and all sorts. It was a link to an article that was posted in 2017 and there did seem to be something maybe to it. It was a small study, the usual limitations, but I couldn't find anything directly naysaying it yet. When I looked into it further, he was talking and explaining some of the symptoms that were on my original list that no one ever looked at. I thought, oh, well, if they're on his list too, maybe it's worth a punt ...

LIVING WITH LONG-TERM CONDITIONS: REFLECTIONS AND RESPONSES TO THESE STORIES

Immediate questions

1. What connections are there between physical and mental ill health in these stories?
2. What ways could the NHS provide psychological support to people like Katie, who have lived with a debilitating condition for so many years?
3. What is the value of the networks of family and friends for people living with long-term conditions?
4. These five stories tell of very different experiences of the support and care given by GPs. How can GP surgeries organise care better around the needs of people who live with long-term health conditions, and what difference might that make?

Strategic questions

1. Recent research suggests that lupus patients like Jasmin, from black and Asian minority ethnic groups, suffer more serious complications than others (Maningding et al., 2019). How can healthcare professionals develop better awareness of how

people from different ethnic backgrounds might be differently affected by their long-term condition?

2. How can healthcare professionals build trust, confidence and parity in their relationships with patients living with long-term conditions?

3. What are the particular needs of patients who have diagnosed or undiagnosed rare conditions?

4. What role do private medicine and complementary therapies play in these stories? What could the NHS learn from these services to improve the help it provides for people living with challenging long-term health conditions?

5. What is the role of self-help and support groups and what are their limitations, according to these stories?

REFERENCES

Demain, S., A.C. Gonçalves, C. Areia, R. Oliveira, A.J. Marcos, A. Marques, R. Parmar and K. Hunt (2015) "Living with, managing and minimising treatment burden in long term conditions: a systematic review of qualitative research", *PLoS One* 10 (5): e0125457.

Maningding, E., M. Dall'Era, L. Turpin, L. Murphy and J. Yazdany (2019) "Racial/ethnic differences in prevalence of and time to onset of SLE manifestations: the California Lupus Surveillance Project (CLSP)", *Arthritis Care and Research* 7 (5): 622–629.

King's Fund (2013) "Long-term conditions and multi-morbidity", Time to Think Differently Project, www.kingsfund.org.uk/projects/time-think-differently/trends-disease-and-disability-long-term-conditions-multi-morbidity (accessed 5 January 2021).

NHS (2014) *Five Year Forward View*, www.england.nhs.uk/wp-content/uploads/2014/10/5yfv-web.pdf (accessed 3 January 2021).

❧ 5 ❧

ADULT ACUTE CARE
AND CANCER

INTRODUCTION

Urgent and emergency care (by which we mean a procedure which needs to be done immediately) is, by its very nature, different from planned care. The diagnosis is not always easy to nail down: the patient might be in considerable pain, distress or shock, and the trajectory of care can be uncertain. Cancer care raises issues (and a set of policies) of its own. One of the most high-profile targets in the NHS, introduced in 2000, is the four-hour waiting time target for patients to be seen, treated, transferred or discharged in A&E departments. The target resulted, in the early years, in huge drops in the number of long waits. Since 2011, performance against this target has steadily deteriorated across all hospitals in England, with some patients waiting over twelve hours on trolleys and in corridors (Nuffield Trust, 2020). New proposals are designed to measure the average waiting time for patients in A&E departments, as a less blunt and more realistic assessment of timely care.

Demand on the ambulance service and on emergency hospital beds has steadily increased in recent years. This trend correlates with the increase in the numbers of frail older people as well as growth in the general population. However, it is likely that the increase in demand is affected by changes in the funding and organisation of services as well as by numbers of patients. Policies to avoid acute hospital admissions, with schemes to provide "care closer to home", helplines such as NHS 111 and the provision of urgent treatment centres have had variable impacts. The emergency care system continues to be under strain, especially during winter, and increasingly (and even before COVID-19) all year round.

Planned care is also subject to targets in the English NHS. Patients should not wait longer than eighteen weeks for non-urgent, consultant-led treatments. As with emergency care, the NHS has increasingly struggled to meet this target in recent years, with many people enduring delays in getting the operation, procedure or investigation done. Some specialties remain more problematic in relation to timely access to treatment than others. The NHS Long Term Plan (NHS, 2019) promised additional capacity for a higher volume of planned acute care, including an increased number of hospital beds and staffing to reduce the lengthening waiting lists for diagnostics and operations. Meanwhile, the response of the NHS to the COVID-19 pandemic was to postpone vast swathes of planned care and it remains to be seen whether and to what extent commitments in the Long Term Plan will be honoured. More generally the disruptive effects of COVID-19 have prompted thinking about the need to "reset" the organisation of services, with potentially much longer-term implications, as illustrated by the position statement made by the Royal College of Emergency Medicine (2020).

Cancer services have benefited from the introduction of cancer-specific targets to reduce waiting times for diagnosis and treatment. More people are living for longer after a cancer diagnosis. This success brings new challenges for the provision of appropriate care and support from the local NHS and voluntary sector. Cancer is both an urgent health problem, with significant psychological impacts, and also an illness with longer-term risks and implications for those who have had a cancer diagnosis, and these have to be monitored carefully. As with other types of acute hospital care, cancer services have increasingly struggled to meet targets in recent years, and were to a considerable extent put on hold during the height of the COVID-19 pandemic.

Acute hospital care can be complex; for example, services are often provided by clinical staff from different professions and employed by different organisations, as they hand patients over along the care pathway, and this is illustrated in some of the accounts contained in this chapter. Hospitals themselves are large and complex organisations. Policymakers and professionals have devoted much attention in recent years to how acute care can be delivered more safely, to a higher quality and in more coordinated, patient-centred ways. The Royal College of Physicians' Future Hospital Programme (Royal College of Physicians, 2017) is a case in point, as are the various responses that followed the investigations of failures at the Mid Staffordshire NHS Foundation Trust and in other trusts (Department of Health, 2013).

As with other aspects of healthcare, there is evidence of considerable inequalities in the delivery of acute care. For example, the charity

Mencap has long drawn attention to poor care received by people with learning disabilities and believes that about 1,200 people could be dying avoidably every year as a result. Their document *Treat Me Well* (Mencap, 2017) reviews the evidence and policy developments, and the campaigning that Mencap has led over several years, since its seminal report *Death by Indifference* (Mencap, 2007).

THE STORIES

In Chapter 1 (Section 2, p. 4) we offer an understanding of patient-centred care in general as:

- Understanding and valuing what matters to patients
- Seeing the whole person
- Respecting people's rights and autonomy
- Being customer focussed

Against these criteria, the stories below can be seen as presenting very much a mixed picture.

This chapter contains four stories in which hospital was a significant site for care. The stories cover planned care, emergency care and a story about cancer. The first story is about what happened to **Jill** following an accident involving her knee, including her follow-up care. This is the longest story in the chapter. The second is about a planned operation to remove **Andrea**'s gallbladder. The third concerns **Lucy**'s experience when she was hospitalised with sepsis. The final story concerns **Shona**'s journey to recovery from breast cancer, and what helped along the way. In addition, it is worth cross-referring to Justin and Lucinda's story about **Jim** in Chapter 3, which spans several decades and includes episodes of acute adult care. As with other chapters, we have posed questions at the end arising from these stories, to simulate your thinking and reflection.

Story 12: Jill

While getting ready to go out on a Saturday evening in November, Jill had an accident at home in the bathroom, and badly injured her knee (dislocation of joint and complete tear of ligaments). She waited on the floor of her bathroom for two hours for an ambulance to take her to hospital. She describes how bewildering and lost it can feel to be waiting in an emergency department at night in severe pain. She had an X-ray and an MRI scan and two separate procedures involving a general anaesthetic, to reset the knee and then to repair the ligaments, and went home five days later. Jill experienced very different levels of care and attention in the various wards and departments of the hospital. Her post-operative care was chaotic – the GP surgery explained that they couldn't offer wound care, despite Jill having been steered to them by the hospital, and the hospital did not make contact to arrange follow-up appointments with the surgeon and with the physiotherapist as promised. Jill herself organised all her follow-up care. Despite the potentially catastrophic nature of the injury, following a strict physiotherapy regime, Jill eventually regained 98 per cent function in her damaged knee.

Jill: Well, what happened was I was getting ready to go out for the evening and I stepped into the shower to just get a bottle of shampoo. I was intending to have a bath and as I stepped out of the shower, one foot was on the bath mat and the other foot was in the shower and there was a terrible pain in my knee and I fell. I fell on the floor and the angle of the bottom half of my leg was not right. It was absolutely agonising pain so I screamed and so my husband came tearing up the stairs and I had fallen on the floor slightly behind the bathroom door and I said, phone an ambulance, I think I might have broken my leg. Basically, the bath mat slid away and, as it turned out, I had dislocated my left knee.

So I was lying on the floor, not wearing anything. It was November so it wasn't particularly warm and I live in a rambling Victorian house, but since there was hot water under the floor it wasn't particularly cold. My husband phoned an ambulance. I could hear him phoning. To start with he found it quite difficult to get in the room because I'd fallen just behind the door but then he squeezed in and put a dressing gown over the top of me. I rather assumed that an ambulance would be there fairly quickly and although it was absolute agony – I was crying in pain – that they would give me morphine and it would be all right, but it was a Saturday evening and I fell at 18:20. I was not top priority for the ambulance so it took two hours for an ambulance to get to me.

For all of that time I was lying on the floor and I didn't dare eat or drink anything and I didn't dare take painkillers because I thought at any moment an ambulance would be there. We called and they said, there are other people that are a higher priority, you know. Are you bleeding? I was but not very much. I can see, if an older person's fallen and is having a heart attack, they're going to be higher priority but it was absolute agony. It was excruciating pain and I was there until, I don't know, about 20:30.

God, how awful.

J: It really was just terrible pain ... we phoned a couple of times and they said, yes, you are on the list, you know, if it gets any worse, phone us back. I was literally screaming and crying in pain. Then eventually the ambulance came and the crew were brilliant and they did give me morphine but it didn't stop it hurting. It was still excruciating. They said, she's going to be at least in overnight, will you pack a bag? And they wrapped me up in my dressing gown and they said, can you walk? I just couldn't. I couldn't. I just couldn't stand the pain. So, yes, they put me on this chair thing that they bumped down the stairs which was excruciating and then put me in an ambulance and took me to hospital. My husband came in the car and was with me and I had had morphine but it just didn't touch the pain. A&E was very busy and I was on a trolley for quite a long time and eventually then I was put in a room.

The pain was still excruciating but A&E was rammed. The woman from the ambulance crew stayed quite a while with me because I wasn't going anywhere. I was just in the corridor. My husband kept going to the nurses and asking could I have any more pain relief and they gave me paracetamol or something and at some point they topped up the morphine but they didn't actually do anything until 02:30 in the morning. By which time A&E had cleared out a bit with people in hand-cuffs and the police. There was quite a lot of that going on.

At some point they X-rayed it I think. I was waiting quite a long time at X-ray and then they told me that I had dislocated it and that it wouldn't stop hurting until they essentially realigned it but they couldn't do that yet. They would need to give me a general anaesthetic to do that. I kept saying but the pain is awful and they kept saying, yes, we know the pain is awful but we can't really do anything until we realign it. So at 02:30 my husband eventually went home because I said, look, they're going to give me a general anaesthetic, there isn't any point in you being here, go home. He wouldn't go before that because I was just in such dreadful pain. He didn't want to leave me. Although they'd given me more morphine it hadn't really helped. Well, it had helped a little. I wasn't actually screaming. I was just sobbing quietly.

Maybe I should have made more of a fuss, I don't know. When they reset it, I woke up and my leg was in almost a box of plaster with some kind of elastic gauze over the top, that held it there, but I was lying down with three sides of plaster round it. They said, yes, they'd reset it and they gave me more morphine and eventually they took me up to a ward to wait for a bed to be available for me. Then I tried to phone my mum and I tried to phone my husband because I had my mobile with me. Then they offered me, I don't know, tea and toast or something and because I've lived here twenty-five years now and I've taught a lot of children, I know a lot of people and one of the occupational therapists who came through the ward was someone I knew. I taught her children. There was an incident with the child which meant that I knew the mum very well, so she said, oh, would you like a cup of tea? She came and sat with me and chatted. That was really nice because everyone was so busy, you know, nobody had a chance to talk or to tell you what was going on or where you were going to end up.

I tried to phone my mum and there was a cleaner hoovering so she couldn't hear me, so then she tried to phone me back and I couldn't hear her because the hoover was going. So that was really quite difficult because I hadn't told Mum. I didn't want to worry her, but then eventually I managed to talk to her and then that morning, I was taken up to a ward which dealt with knees and hips, basically, mostly elective [planned] surgery.

They were not as busy as either the ward I was on temporarily that morning or A&E because in the run-up to Christmas, I believe that people hadn't elected to have their surgery. So they were less busy than other places might be. Also, because I'd had a stomach upset that day before I fell, they didn't want to put me with everybody else. They wanted to put me in a room by myself in case my stomach upset went elsewhere, I think. I had this lovely room with its own en-suite with a beautiful view and the staff were absolutely lovely and they did have time because they weren't busy, so after that it was good.

So that would have been on the Sunday I went to the ward, and I think to start with there was the issue of using the loo and the bed pan and could I get up? No, I couldn't. Oh, and I had to have another imaging thing and it wasn't an X-ray because the X-ray was, I'm trying to remember, good for bones but not very good for soft tissue.

So at some point on the Monday I went downstairs and had this scan and then they looked at it and said that they were considering the options on what to do about the knee. Then late on Monday evening a nice doctor, not the consultant but one of his team, came to see me and said, right, then, Mrs X ... You know, there's no point me saying Ms because they just don't deal with Ms, really. I've always been Ms X ... but, hey, the national health doesn't get that.

So anyway, we will need to operate on your knee. You've been told you're having an operation in the morning? No, nobody's told me that. Oh, haven't they? Oh, well, you are having an operation in the morning. Okay, why am I having an operation in the morning? Well, you have torn all the ligaments in your knee and you need ligaments in your knee for it to work, so basically we've got to create ligaments so that your knee works again. What happened in the early hours of Sunday morning was just putting the knee joint in place but we need to put ligaments in place otherwise it won't work. I'm afraid you'll probably have a limp. Now, I didn't think that was a big problem, really. I'd had, what I saw as an absolutely excruciating fall. I'd had breast cancer six years ago.

I was delighted to be cancer-free. Having a limp seemed small beer. It wasn't like it was going to interfere with my international footballing career. I wondered why he was worried about it, really, but he seemed to be terribly worried that I might have a limp. I mean, at 54, how big a deal is that, really? Anyway, so the next day I did have the surgery. The surgeon was very pleased with himself. Everyone told me, all the nurses told me he was a very, very good surgeon. Yes, he had been to see me before the operation and told me that he was going to create ligaments. He was, kind of, like Jeff Goldblum, if some kind of person like that exists, and he was charming and smooth and very confident in his own abilities.

Did that annoy you?

J: No, it didn't. I think if you're going to have surgery, it's quite a good idea to have someone who seems to know what they're doing. So, no, it didn't annoy me. I thought he was handsome and charming, which is never a bad thing. Not necessarily someone I would have wanted to go out with at the age of 20, but the sort of person that you might like to do your surgery at the age of 54.

I did mention to the anaesthetist that he was like Jeff Goldblum and he said, oh, for God's sake, don't tell him that, he's arrogant enough already. So anyway, the surgery was done and when I woke up, I was back in the ward and I didn't have the plaster on anymore. I had some other contraption on my leg and it was all bandaged up and, yes, I was getting up and using the loo and it was awkward. I had a walking frame to do that and the nurses were terribly helpful, you know. They were really good. Yes, so it was fine and the physiotherapists were brilliant but I had to keep taking the morphine because if the pain broke through it was still considerable.

The morphine made me sick. The physiotherapists talked about me going home fairly quickly. They wouldn't let me go home until I had mastered the stairs with crutches, well, with a crutch, because there's an order you have to do the stairs in terms of good foot, walking aid, bad foot, up and down the stairs. Until I had done that, they wouldn't let me go. I thought I wanted to go home and they talked about me going home on Thursday, which was quite quick, really, but on Thursday I became less confident about that because I felt so sick. Every time I got up to do the physiotherapist's bidding I felt terribly sick and had to come and sit down again. Late in the day, one of the nurses said, I'm not sure you should go today, but then we'd made arrangements and I thought, oh, I think I'd better go for it, really. So I did go home on Thursday. At the advice of the physiotherapists some friends had moved a bed downstairs for me because we have a loo downstairs, so that I didn't have to climb the stairs for bed because I was just exhausted by going to the toilet.

That wasn't very good, really, because what we hadn't considered was that a hospital bed is really high and this particular bed that was brought down was quite low and had a memory foam mattress so was hell on earth to get out of because it was so low. By that time I had no bandage on my leg but I had this contraption, a splint thing with Velcro on and it had a knee joint and to start with I was not to move my leg more than 10 degrees.

I had to keep it very stiff. There were staples in and stitches in, so, yes, that was really difficult so I only spent two nights in that bed because I didn't like it. I didn't like being away from my husband and he didn't like me being away from him because he felt if I needed anything he couldn't hear me and our bed is much higher, so I just had to do the stairs. Then he wasn't happy going to work and leaving me with the stairs to do, so, yes, we had to make arrangements, really.

The biggest NHS problem I had after that was after so many days I needed to have the staples and stitches out and they said the surgery would do that but the surgery couldn't do that. They didn't have the capacity to do it. As it happened, one of the nurses was off because her father had died so they couldn't do it and they said, go to the walk-in centre.

Now, as it happens, our walk-in centre is closing next month so I don't know what people will do then, but that's another matter. I felt the walk-in centre was not ideal: I can't walk, or very few steps. So what I did was I phoned a friend who, oddly enough, I had texted when I was lying on the floor, because she's a district nurse, to ask her if there was anything I could do to stop the excruciating pain given that I'd been waiting an hour and a half for an ambulance. Then she messaged me when she got the text which was later on. She'd come to see me in hospital and had said, you know, if you have any trouble getting the stitches out, let me know and I'll come and do it for you.

So she did that for me. I'm very reluctant to march in and say, hello, I am the chair of the patient participation group [PPG] and you really should get my stitches out. That would seem terribly arrogant and some-body was off sick for a perfectly good reason, but I was very disappointed that the surgery said they couldn't take my stitches out.

I was lucky that I had someone who could do it for me at home. What about all the people who aren't lucky? I thought that was a bit of a fail, really.

Yes, so then I did have to nag because I was supposed to have a follow-up appointment and nothing happened. I was supposed to have physi-otherapy, nothing happened. So I phoned the surgeon's secretary and she said, oh, you should have had it by now. Can you come in this afternoon? There was then a bit of a panic. Can you come now? Well, obviously I couldn't drive. I did go and then there was the same thing with the physiotherapy. That didn't materialise. I was supposed to have physiotherapy and, again, I phoned the surgeon's secretary and said, you know you sorted the follow-up appointment, well, the physiotherapy hasn't happened either. She said, oh, no, I'm so sorry it's gone wrong again and then I got a call the next morning to say, can you come in now for physiotherapy?

Very last minute and I said, well, no, I'm going to a funeral this morning. I can't, no. Oh, well, you'll have to wait two weeks then. Well, I should have had physiotherapy by then. So that was hopeless, but when I actually did get to see the physiotherapist she was, you know, as they usually are, physio-terrorists, and was very fierce.

Physio-terrorist!

J: Well, they cause you pain, don't they? Have you never had physiotherapy?

Yes, I have and it can be quite painful.

J: They cause you pain, don't they? No gain without pain. You have to and I honestly did what I was told though it bloody hurt. She told me I couldn't possibly go to Venice for Christmas. So I guess it couldn't have been that long because I saw her just before Christmas, I think. I went anyway. She said you'll never get travel insurance and I phoned the travel insurance and they said, yes, it's fine. To be honest, it wasn't ideal going to Venice with two crutches but I had arranged things so that it was okay and it was actually easier being in an apart-ment in Venice which was all on one floor than being in my house at home. The physiotherapy was very good. I did it very earnestly and as a result, when I had my annual check in November, I've got 98 per cent of the movement back in my leg, which they didn't expect me to get.

That's really good. Do you have a limp?

J: No. Well, I do if I get very tired. The only thing I find difficult … Well, there are two things, really. One is if I go down a steep hill, I feel it afterwards in that knee. So it looks ridiculous when I do it but I live at the top of a very steep hill, I go down sideways which looks ridiculous but means I don't hurt afterwards. The other thing is getting up off the floor because I can't kneel on it. Well, I can if it's the bed but other than that I can't. In that case, I tend do a, sort of, downward-facing dog, if you know what I mean, to get up and that works. So I can get up and down. It looks awkward but it works. Other than that I don't run because the surgeon told me I mustn't.

The only running I ever do is in aqua-aerobics. I can do a forty-five-minute aqua-aerobics class without a problem. I try to avoid the jumping bits because that doesn't feel good. Sometimes it aches a bit afterwards, but it's all right, actually.

I mean I think lessons learned might be, you know, should it really take more than two hours to get an ambulance?

It would be quite nice to tell the patient what you're going to do to them before you do to them.

It would be nice if the appointment system worked so if the ward are going to organise the follow-up and the physiotherapy it'd be good if they actually did. Yes, and it would be good if the surgery had the capacity to do the things that the hospital say they're going to do. I've since found, being on the PPG, that wound dressing is an absolute nightmare for surgeries. Hospitals assume they have the capacity and they don't necessarily. So I think that's quite a big issue that runs across a lot of areas.

It does sound as though all your interactions with health professionals were pretty good but a lot of the organisation and admin and communication was terrible.

J: Yes, absolutely. The nurses I had in hospital were darlings, absolutely brilliant, even the student nurses were really good. In fact, I've stayed in contact with one of them. Fantastic, they were absolutely brilliant, the staff in the hospital – apart from whoever was supposed to organise the appointments afterwards. The physiotherapists were great, were very sympathetic but pushed you. Yes, I mean the fact of the matter is – they didn't tell me this until afterwards – I had a catastrophic injury which could have been so much worse and I have 98 per cent of my movement back. Now, that is a result.

Yes.

J: To some extent, is it only because I knew the system well enough to know who to phone to get action fairly quickly?

Yes, I was going to say, and you said it yourself, that there were parts of this experience where it really helped to know the system and other people would not have had that advantage.

J: Absolutely, I mean, at some point, I was a drugs rep for [a large pharmaceutical company], so I know that phoning the secretary of the person is the thing to do, to get your way through the system.

Yes, that's interesting. The other thing, I mean, was your pain managed properly or was it inevitable that you were going to be in extreme pain that they couldn't do much about?

J: Well, that's an interesting case. I don't know, honestly. When I was in A&E the pain was excruciating. Talking to my friend who was the district nurse who came and removed my staples, she said that she had concerns that since they've reorganised the ambulance service, the people prioritising didn't necessarily have the medical knowledge to prioritise and that some injuries were left because they weren't seen as a priority but could have been disastrous if they were left too long. So, for example, I was a bit frightened by a couple of newspaper reports I read after that, where I saw that somebody with similar injuries had lost their leg because they had waited too long and they had got compartment syndrome and therefore lost the leg.

I was very fortunate. One of the things they seemed to be concerned about was, did I have blood flow to the bottom of my leg because I'd severed the ligaments but I don't think I'd damaged the blood vessel. If I had, I think things might have been rather different.

I don't have enough medical knowledge to know that but because they were concerned about the blood flow, I suspect that might have been an issue but they didn't know that before they'd turned up in the ambulance.

No, and that wasn't a question they were asking on the phone, then, was it, about whether you could feel your toes?

J: No, well, they asked if I was bleeding and I had just hit my calf on the lip of the shower as I went down so it wasn't bad at all. It wasn't even bad enough to need a plaster, really. The crucial point was the dislocation: I was lying on my side on the floor on the good leg with the bad leg on top, well, slightly at an angle, partially on top.

Yes, for two hours. Dreadful.

J: It was. It was something I would never want to repeat. It was excruciating pain. I have never had pain like it, mind you, I had two caesareans, but it was excruciating. The pain was managed in hospital. They gave me, I suppose it was Oramorph which I liked very much. It tasted like Bakewell tarts and you could feel it kicking in. Your head started floating. So the pain went, of course it caused other things, made you feel sick, terrible constipation but other than that … So once I got out of hospital I didn't take it anymore. I took co-codamol. They gave me a packet of morphine and I never took it because I didn't want to feel sick and be constipated, really.

Is there anything else about that experience that you think is worth sharing?

J: The follow-up appointments: first one was with the surgeon and he was pleased with the progress. The second two were with part of his team and they were all very efficient, they were all very charming and praised my extensive efforts at physiotherapy so I felt like I'd done something good. Everyone likes to be praised so, yes, they did well. I didn't have to wait long for my appointments.

Story 13: Andrea

Andrea had an operation to remove her gallbladder. She went to her doctor's surgery with symptoms of pain and vomiting; the doctor provisionally diagnosed gallstones (which proved correct) and sent her for a scan. The GP promptly called her back into the surgery after the scan result to arrange a hospital outpatient appointment, explaining that an operation would be needed. She explains how well coordinated the care was, including the flow of appointments and follow-ups at the GP surgery, the local NHS hospital which carried out the scan, the health centre where the hospital consultant ran an outpatient clinic, and the private hospital where the operation took place. She was surprised to find herself as an NHS patient being treated in a private hospital.

Andrea did not know that her GP surgery has an Outstanding rating with the Care Quality Commission.

So, what happened at the beginning? I understand you had a gallbladder operation. How did it first manifest itself that you had a problem? And particularly what happened when you first went to the GP?

Andrea: A serious amount of pain in the night, which made me feel ... well made me sick ... went to the GP. They recognised straightaway what it was, got me a scan booked.

So, they got the right diagnosis.

A: They knew the tell-tale signs for what they thought it was.

How did you feel about that, that the GP got to the diagnosis so quickly?

A: Pleased. Very, very pleased, because you never just know what it could be. I got the scan appointment within three weeks, which was before Christmas. Went for the scan, they said that, yes, that I had got gallstones, but I would hear from my GP. Between Christmas and the New Year, I got a telephone call off my GP to say could I make an appointment to go down and see them. Which I did do, I saw my GP before New Year. I went into the surgery, and the doctor brought it all up on the computer. They told me obviously I needed to have an operation, and they booked me an appointment there and then with the consultant, to see him middle to end of January. And they actually booked me an appointment online at the health centre in a local town, when the consultant was there.

And presumably at a date and a time that was also convenient for you?

A: They asked me what day and what time would be convenient for me.

So, how did you feel about how the GP organised the care for you? Because he or she basically had to refer you and then got the results and then referred you on to the consultant.

A: Really, really pleased. They were just on the ball. There was no, oh, it'll be a waiting list. You put your trust in them and they just did it for you.

So, which hospital did you go to for your operation?

A: XXX, which is a private hospital. Which I was really quite shocked about, but as long as it got my problem sorted, I wasn't bothered where I went.

So, tell me why you were shocked about that?

A: Because I just thought I'd be going into a normal NHS hospital. Not a privately run hospital.

Was it explained why you were referred there?

A: No, it wasn't actually, no.

It wasn't explained by the GP?

A: No.

Was it explained by the doctor at the hospital or anyone else?

A: No. They just said, there you go, you've got a place at the private hospital.

So, you went for an outpatient appointment there? And what happened then?

A: I went and saw the consultant at the health centre in the local town, because the consultant works at the local NHS hospital and he works at the private hospital as well.

So, you didn't have to go to the private hospital for the outpatient appointment?

A: No. The only time I had to go there was to have a swab done for MRSA. That was the only time I had to go, I had to have that done about ten days before I went in for my operation. But no, they made the appointment for me at the local health centre to see the consultant. I saw him, he was brilliant, explained absolutely everything that was going to happen. He gave you confidence that he knew everything was going to go according to plan.

Okay, so you had the operation and were you discharged on the same day?

A: Yes.

And then, how was the care after the operation organised for you? Or did you not need any care?

A: I was told I couldn't lift anything, or anything like that, and then they made me an appointment there and then at the hospital to see the consultant after six weeks.

And did you have to go back to the private hospital for that, or did you go to the local health centre?

A: I had to go to the health centre in the local town, where they made the appointment.

And is that convenient for you where you live?

A: Yes. It's not too bad.

*Is it more convenient than the private hospital?***A:**Yes, definitely.

And did you have any other aftercare? Did the district nurse need to come or anything like that?

A: No, but I did go down to my local surgery because I had a slight problem with one of the wounds, it wasn't healing correctly. So, I went and saw the nurses at my GP's, and they sorted it out for me. And then they told me to go down again and see them again to make sure that everything was healing correctly.

And how easy was it to see the nurse?

A: Yeah, fine. Just rang up and I think I had to wait a day to see the practice nurse.

So, all in all, in terms of how the care was organised, what do you say might be the learning for the NHS?

A: It was just so quick; they knew exactly what to do … when to do it … and it just flowed.

Did that surprise you?

A: Yeah.

Tell me why.

A: Because I thought I was going to have to wait months and months and months even to see a consultant. I didn't think it was going to flow as easily as what it did. With what I've heard with other people, having to wait months and months and months. I was really, really shocked.

Story 14: Lucy

Lucy lives with a serious long-term mental illness. Her experiences of mental health services are described in Chapter 6. She is a consultant psychiatrist. Here she describes, after an initial visit to A&E resulted in the wrong diagnosis because of her chronic kidney disease, what happened when she got hospitalised with sepsis. First she was taken to the medical assessment ward, and then on to a ward for older people over 75. After that she ended up on a post-operative gynaecology ward. There was a huge difference in how well Lucy felt cared for in this last ward. She was upset about how badly managed the ward for older people was and it had a negative effect on both her physical health and her mental well-being.

Lucy: When I retired, I was diagnosed with chronic kidney disease … which turns out that I've had all my life, but it's just been getting gradually worse. I've always had problems with persistent urinary tract infections [UTIs] and I got a persistent UTI and bleeding and I was investigated and I was found to have polycystic kidney disease. And my renal function is okay, but it's very slowly deteriorating, because it's come to notice late, whereas for some people, it comes to notice when they're in their 20s and 30s. I don't know if I'll ever need to go on dialysis, but it's a possibility.

So I'm under the care of the regional unit in XXX and one of the problems is that XXX hospital can't see YYY hospital's data … they can only see the reports; they can't see the actual images, because one of them is an academic organisation … they can't see each other's ultrasounds, and it's ridiculous, and this has gone on … Last year, I had some bleeding and I saw my GP, and the XXX [hospital] thought it might be a burst cyst. And then I went for investigations. And five days after I had the cystoscopy done, I developed a terrible pain and vomiting. And we went up to A&E on the Monday morning, and it was a bank holiday, so

I went through all of the NHS Direct and I knew they were going to say, go to A&E, so I did.

And they thought it might be a burst cyst again, because I didn't have a high temperature, but sent me home with some codeine, and I was better for a few hours, and then on the next day, I was lying on the sofa and I just got worse all day, until about eight o'clock in the evening, when I really felt like I was dying. They took one look at me at reception and said, you can go straight through, because I was actually vomiting at reception, so they didn't like that. And the team in A&E were absolutely great, they actually diagnosed sepsis straightaway.

I had a high temperature, my blood pressure was falling, my urine electrolytes, when they got them back, were all over the place, my liver function tests were starting to go off, and the registrar was absolutely great. He just said, it's sepsis. They stuck a needle in both arms and catheterised me, and that was that. But then I went to the medical assessment unit and I lay on a trolley for about an hour, but I did get a bed, and then I saw a couple of people there who took my history again and they kept putting lots of fluids into me and they started me on antibiotics. But then the next step was awful. The only bed they could find was on an older person's ward, for over 75s, and they said they had a bed, but when we went up there, the person hadn't left their bed and I was left sitting in a chair with no headrest for two hours, and I was acutely ill, and [my partner] was with me and I had my head sort of just leaning against him.

And the ward was just awful. It was dirty and the auxiliary staff were a bit out of control … I've been an auxiliary nurse, as a student, so I know they were running the place. And they were not very nice people and they made a mistake with my medication one night and they gave me oral instead of intravenous, and I knew they had. And I was a bit out of it for the first couple of days, and they would come and get you out of bed in the morning and make you sit next to the bed until they remade the bed, which was like two hours, and I was really ill and it was horrible. Anyway, after a week, they needed that bed for someone who was more ill, so they moved me to a gynae ward, post-surgical, and that was completely different. That was run and organised like a ward when I was a medical student. It had a sister who came round to check if everything was all right, and they came round in the morning and they said, would you like us to refresh your bed, and they did, and I was able to get out and get straight back in. People came and did everything at the right time.

I'd had these cannulas in for days and they were filthy, and she took them out, and they should have been changed after forty-eight hours, but I was too ill to argue. And so I had good care there, and I thought, it's really interesting, this is a surgical ward, and I know surgeons are more powerful than medics ... There were some very sick people there, who were also old. The woman opposite me had to go back to theatre because she was really going downhill, and I thought, it's about the power of surgeons, this is.

Do you think that's what it was?

L: I think surgeons are much better at getting what they want in hospitals than medics are. I never found out in the older persons ward which team was looking after me. Nobody ever said, we are looking after you. There was a succession of doctors who never introduced themselves. No one said, hello, my name is ... except for the nurse on the acute medical unit, and then they did when I went to the other ward. It was chaos and it was poorly managed and no one seemed to be in charge of the place. The beds on the older person's ward were horrible, they were hard. Once I got to the other ward, it was possible to sleep in them without having to put a pillow under my hip.

What about the nurses, though? Because it's not all about the doctors, is it?

L: I just felt they weren't managed. I think it was a management failure. When I spoke to the chief executive, he emailed back to say that they were not short-staffed on that ward; he said it was almost certainly a management issue. I don't think they were running the place properly.

They've apparently got a home IV service, but it's so underfunded that they couldn't get me onto it, so I spent an extra four or five days in hospital. Having had all of those investigations at the XXX the week before I went in there, I had to have them all again because they couldn't see the ones that had been done at there. So I had ultrasound again. I'd even had an MRI scan at the XXX but that couldn't be seen. But all of that had to be repeated, even though all the investigations had been done, you know, a week before.

So how long were you in altogether? Nearly two weeks?

L: Two weeks.

And how did that affect your mental health? Did it have an effect on your mental health?

L: Well, I got very down. Well, I was quite confused for a couple of days. And I thought there was an underground station in the ward at one point.

An underground station?

L: Yeah, I could hear trains and things. It was all very weird. And then I got a bit down because I was in persistent pain and they kept just wanting to give me paracetamol and that wasn't working. And there was a point where I felt quite down and I thought … I've had patients who have thrown themselves out of windows in hospital wards before now. I thought, I can understand how they do it, because if people are really being vile to you, you just reach a point where you think, I'll go out the window. But once I got over to the other ward, I started to cheer up a bit. And I stopped one of my antidepressants because I couldn't cope with swallowing it, and the nurses kept trying to give it to me, and they said, oh, we don't want you to go funny! So I actually rang up my consultant. I emailed him, because I could email by then, and he rang me. He was at the Isle of Wight Festival; I think he was into heavy metal in his youth, or something … He said, are you sure you want to stop them? And I said, yes, and he said, all right then.

So I didn't have any withdrawal symptoms, or if I did, I couldn't tell because I'd got so much else going on. But my blood pressure just wouldn't come up and I was worried that that was making it worse. They kept coming and wanting to take my blood pressure very frequently because it was so low …

How do you think staff treat you differently when you have a physical illness, when they know you have a diagnosis of a mental illness as well?

L: I think they treat you with kid gloves, and I know, from talking to people whom I've met and whom I've treated, that very often they don't want anything to do with them because they've got a mental illness … They don't want to have to deal with the difficulties. They don't want to have to have the negotiation that you sometimes have to have. So I can think of my patients, you know … I had a patient that had an abnormal cervical smear and had bipolar disorder, and just trying to get her to the clinic was really hard. She didn't want to go because of the way people talked to her there. And then when they get there, people often just confound that by not treating her very nicely because they know she's got a mental illness and she might be a bit difficult.

And I've got a friend who has severe mental illness and who has terrible problems because they really don't take into account the fact that
they might need to spend more time with her and she might have these
fears, and anxiety might make her other problems worse, so they get
impatient. When I was starting to get quite down and a bit irritable with
them, over the pain, I could sense they really didn't want to know.

*And why is that? I mean, because nurses and doctors have, as part of their
training, they do have training in mental health, don't they?*

L: A lot of general nurses don't get very much training, and I do think
there's a lot of things about how people often view mental health problems as bad behaviour, I really do. Even mental health nurses do that.
Something that's under your control, you know, you can stop it.

   If you're psychotic, it's like, oh well, you're really mad, you know, you
can't control it … But if you're not psychotic, then it's just you, it's just
you being difficult. Some of the people I've spoken to over the years
have had awful experiences with physical health problems because of
that.

In the sense that they don't feel they're on their side or they're not listened to?

L: They don't feel they're listened to. They feel that they're just treated
as difficult and troublesome. That's one of the reasons why people with
self-injury get treated so badly in A&E, because it's treated as bad behaviour, they're a nuisance, and some of them just don't get good treatment. Well, terrible treatment.

*And why do you think that some of the healthcare staff put that, and particularly
mental health staff, put that nuisance label on people?*

L: Because it's easy. It means you don't have to actually sit down with
people and try and understand why they're feeling …

Story 15: Shona

Shona has had breast cancer. Shona had positive experiences when
first diagnosed and treated, including kindness shown by the nurses
during chemotherapy treatment. She has been on long-term treatment to prevent recurrence and has suffered significant side effects.
Shona describes how clinicians don't always appear very understanding

of the impact on the patient's quality of life of treatments that are prescribed.

Shona: I was diagnosed with breast cancer in 2012. Three years before that I did find a lump in the same place. I went to see my GP and they referred me to the hospital.

They found that the lump I had was not cancerous, they said, and they took the lump out, but they said, let us know if it comes back again and contact my GP, and that was it. And then two years on, in March, I felt the lump again but I thought it was just tissue which had hardened from the previous operation I'd had. So I went back to my GP and said I was a bit concerned and so she said she'd send me back to the hospital, which she did. They did a tissue biopsy and they found that it was cancerous. I was referred to an oncologist. He said that they would only do a lumpectomy – I thought I would have to have a mastectomy. They checked my lymph nodes and it had gone into my lymph nodes but they didn't know how many. So they scheduled the operation I had the lumpectomy and they took fourteen lymph nodes from under my arm. Only two was actually infected. So I stayed overnight in hospital.

My mum passed away the weekend I had my operation. It was a really tough time. They said I'd have to wait three weeks to start my chemo. I had to have six cycles. Obviously I lost my hair and it was a gruelling time and it is such an awful thing to go through. It really is. Then I waited another three weeks before I started my radiotherapy and was for three weeks, every day except for Saturday and Sunday.

I'm on Tamoxifen tablets now. I was suffering a lot with the side effects. I thought, the five years is up and so I can come off it and go back to some sort of normality. But when I went to my oncologist he said that they are now finding that with a lot of women who have come off it after five years, the cancer comes back. So he's suggested me staying on it for another five years or possibly for life. A lot of my friends who are also on Tamoxifen have also come off it after five years as they are really having a tough time with it.

Does it give you a tough time being on Tamoxifen?

S: I've got used to it now. I would say the first four years were very difficult with the side effects, because I suffer with osteoarthritis. Tamoxifen affects all your joints and muscles, it makes you tired, that sort of thing. It affects people in different ways. But my body has got used to it now. I've been taking this for eight years now so it's in my system.

Do you think that doctors understand enough about what it's like living with quite severe side effects of medication?

S: No, I don't think they do. They have so many patients coming in. Since I was diagnosed, it seems that every other person you speak to has had cancer or knows someone that's going through it. They've been overwhelmed with the amount of people who've been diagnosed. So I don't think they really understand. No matter how you are feeling, they are more concerned about the tablets you are taking rather than you as a person.

And, of course, when you go there you've only got five minutes with them. It's only at the beginning when you are diagnosed that they seem to have more time. After two or three years you're just a normal patient and they have to tick the boxes and in five minutes you're out the door.

The thing is you don't get to see your oncologist, you see his registrar, maybe he's so busy, he doesn't have the time to see you. That is the thing I found difficult, because the first year, you build up this relationship with him but then after the second year if your treatment's gone well and you are sort of on the road to recovery then you're passed on to his registrar. Then you have to go through the whole thing again with them. You don't always see the same person, that's the other thing. They have notes but for some reason they still ask you what happened.

The other thing was, apart from the support that I got from the hospital, the nurses who did the chemo were amazing, they really knew their stuff. They knew what you were going through as well. Obviously they had a lot of patients coming in.

I was also offered physiotherapy after that and I was even offered counselling because my mum had just died. I was also offered the services of a charitable organisation. What happens is when you are diagnosed with any type of cancer they give you six or seven free treatments. You can have reflexology, acupuncture and massage. They teach you about nutrients. And it was amazing, I thought it was such a good idea. So I was offered that. You got a goody bag with lots of makeup and things. It was nice and it gives you a bit of a lift and made you feel you're a woman.

My faith helped me so much. I don't think I'd would've been able to cope without it. Father X was very good and he was such a strength. So I had a lot of family and friends around and gave me a lot of support. And my boss was good as well because I had to have time off, obviously.

It's interesting because some of the most important things that supported you were nothing do with the NHS.

S: You are right, because there were a couple of women who were there with me. One was a lady who was in her near 80s. She didn't have family. A taxi had to bring her in for her to have her chemo and she'd go home very tired and she used to be sick with it and not have anybody there to make her a cup of tea. She said she'd just get into bed and sleep right through to the following day.

In terms of the doctors and nurses and actually all the other people involved, what were some of the things that stood out as really good in your memory?

S: The doctors. I have to say, they're not there now. Apparently they've left, they've retired or have moved on to another hospital. The oncologist I had was amazing; he was such a nice guy. Even the surgeon. I think their support at the beginning, just to make sure that I had the right treatment, and obviously if I wasn't happy about anything I just had to pick up the phone and speak to the nurse. My nurse was very supportive, she was always there if I needed anything. But, like I said, most of the time I just got on with it.

ADULT ACUTE CARE: REFLECTIONS AND RESPONSES TO THESE STORIES

Immediate questions

1. What might have led to the circumstances where follow-up wound care was available at one of the GP surgeries, for Andrea, and not at the other, for Jill?

2. What does Lucy's story suggest about the scope for improvement in the hospital care of patients with mental ill health who are admitted with physical health problems?

3. Why might patients feel good about being praised by their clinician for doing well in their rehabilitation?

4. What do Jill's and Shona's experiences of post-operative follow-up care suggest about the improvements that could be made?

5. Jill was reassured rather than annoyed by her surgeon's self-satisfied manner. Andrea was surprised to be treated in a private hospital as an NHS patient. What do these instances tell us about patients' expectations, and what are the implications for professionals in their communications with patients and their families?

6. Was it necessary for Lucy to undergo repeat tests because of the inability of hospital IT systems to communicate with each other?

Strategic questions
1. What does good-quality care look and feel like, according to these testimonies?
2. What do these stories illuminate about the impact on patients of shorter than expected and longer than expected waits for care?
3. Lucy thought her surgical ward was better run than her medical ward because surgeons are better at getting their way in a hospital than medical doctors. Is that a plausible analysis? What role do power hierarchies play in delivering (or failing to deliver) good care?
4. These stories include instances of people using workarounds or exploiting their contacts or inside knowledge of the NHS to get the care they need. How do you feel about this? What are the implications for equity? How should the NHS respond?
5. What can individual health professionals and managers do to join up care better between hospitals and between hospital, community, primary and social services?
6. Why do you think that the moments of kindness described in these stories are so significant for patients?

REFERENCES

Department of Health (2013) *Patients First and Foremost*, Cm 8576 (London: HMSO), https://assets.publishing.service.gov.uk/government/uploads/system/uploads/attachment_data/file/170701/Patients_First_and_Foremost.pdf (accessed 5 January 2021).

Mencap (2007) *Death by Indifference*, www.basw.co.uk/system/files/resources/basw_121542-4_0.pdf (accessed 5 January 2021).

Mencap (2017) *Treat Me Well* (London: Royal Mencap Society), www.mencap.org.uk/sites/default/files/2018-07/2017.005.01%20Campaign%20report%20digital.pdf (accessed 5 January 2021).

NHS (2019) *The NHS Long Term Plan*, Version 1.2 with corrections, August, www.longtermplan.nhs.uk/wp-content/uploads/2019/08/nhs-long-term-plan-version-1.2.pdf (accessed 3 January 2021).

Nuffield Trust (2020) "Indicators: A&E waiting times", www.nuffieldtrust.
   org.uk/resource/a-e-waiting-times (accessed 5 January 2021).
Royal College of Emergency Medicine (2020) *Position Statement: COVID-19
   resetting emergency department care*, 6 May, www.rcem.ac.uk/docs/
   Policy/RCEM_Position_statement_Resetting_Emergency_Care_
   20200506.pdf (accessed 5 January 2021).
Royal College of Physicians (2017) "Future Hospital Programme: delivering
   the future hospital", RCP programme, 23 November, www.rcplondon.
   ac.uk/projects/outputs/future-hospital-programme-delivering-future-
   hospital (accessed 5 January 2021).

MENTAL HEALTH AND MENTAL ILLNESS

INTRODUCTION

Mental health problems are widespread, at times disabling, yet often hidden. In the UK, nearly half (43.4 per cent) of adults think that they have had a diagnosable mental health condition at some point in their life. One in six (17 per cent) of people over the age of 16 had a common mental health problem in the week prior to being interviewed (Mental Health Foundation, 2016). One in eight (12.8 per cent) of 5- to 19-year-olds had at least one mental disorder when assessed in 2017, and the prevalence of mental disorder among 5- to 15-year-olds has shown a slight increase over time (NHS Digital, 2018).

Since the 1960s, what we would now see as punitive and stigmatising attitudes to "madness", with great reliance on institutional care, have given way to a more community-based, human rights-informed approach. These changes were enabled by the development of new generations of anti-psychotic and mood-stabilising drugs, and spurred on by vocal communities of mental health activists. Societal attitudes to mental illness have also changed, aided by campaigns such as Time to Change (www.time-to-change.org.uk).

Nevertheless, mental health services have not been given the priority awarded to physical health when it comes to staffing, funding and national treatment standards. Access to high-quality, timely and appropriate treatment, whether for anxiety and depression or for more extreme ill health requiring hospitalisation, has been insufficient. There has been growing concern in particular about the widespread mental health problems of children and young people, with demand for services outstripping supply. Recent national policy, as reflected in the

Five Year Forward View for Mental Health (NHS England, 2016) and the NHS Mental Health Implementation Plan (2019), is aimed at boosting provision and reducing the gap between mental and physical health services.

As with other aspects of ill health and organised responses to it, the field of mental health is also marked by deep inequalities. For example, black and minority ethnic people are at higher risk of receiving a diagnosis of mental ill health, and disproportionately impacted by social detriments associated with mental ill health. They can have greater difficulty in accessing appropriate care and support, and have more adverse experiences of assessment and treatment. Black and minority ethnic people are 40 per cent more likely to access mental health services via the criminal justice system than white people. African-Caribbean men are more likely to be diagnosed and hospitalised with schizophrenia and to be detained in secure institutions. The causes of these inequalities are multi-factoral, but discrimination and prejudice play a significant part (Bignall et al., 2019).

THE STORIES

In Chapter 1 (Section 2, p. 4) we offer an understanding of patient-centred care in general as:

- Understanding and valuing what matters to patients
- Seeing the whole person
- Respecting people's rights and autonomy
- Being customer focussed

Against these criteria, the stories below can be seen as presenting very much a mixed picture.

This chapter contains five stories about mental ill health: three from patients, one from a family member, and one from a psychiatrist who is also a patient. We start with **Audrey**, who works as a healthcare scientist and knows how the NHS works. Hers is a fragment of a story, which describes the process of getting access to the right services for her family member. We then move on to **Stanley**, who arrived in the UK from Zimbabwe in 1995 and had his first breakdown and diagnosis of bipolar disorder in 1997. Next comes **Alan**, who has also been living with bipolar disorder for over twenty years and now works as a patient ambassador talking to groups across the country about his experiences. **Nathan** is a teenager with various mental health issues. Finally, **Lucy** provides the longest story in this chapter. She is a retired hospital psychiatrist with lived experience of a severe and enduring mental illness. As with other chapters, we have posed questions at the end, arising from these stories, to simulate your thinking and reflection.

Story 16: Audrey

This is a story fragment about the difficulties encountered by one person in accessing mental health services because they were never quite ill enough or were too ill to fit a particular service. Eventually a family member (who tells this story), with inside knowledge of the NHS, comes to his aid.

Audrey: I have personal experience with a close relative who has suffered for many years with mental health problems and been bounced from one service to another without any kind of effective treatment, being told he was either too severe for one service or not severe enough for the next. After five years, unable to work due to his problems and feeling effectively written off, he did get to see someone, was given a diagnosis and was promised a referral for CBT [cognitive behavioural therapy] but then heard nothing for several months. He is not well enough to chase his own referral, so I did the calling round. When I did, I was told that he was on a waiting list but they could not give me any indication of timescales as to when he would be seen as they had a "huge backlog". They did say they were expecting it to be at least six to eight months before he got to the top of the list and we would not hear anything until then.

It was then that I learned that, unlike in physical health, where patients have the right to be seen and started on treatment within eighteen weeks of referral (and hospitals suffer penalties for failing to meet this target, meaning that huge amounts of resource are diverted to ensuring we meet it), patients with mental health problems have no such right. Concerned about his ever-deteriorating situation, I fought his corner and had to threaten to complain to the CCG [Clinical Commissioning Group] before they suddenly managed to find him an appointment the following week and thankfully, after five years, he is finally starting to turn a corner. I feel very strongly that this is just not right. People suffering from mental health problems are often unable to fight for their rights due to the nature and symptoms of their illness. This does not mean policymakers and the NHS has the right to ignore them.

Story 17: Stanley

Stanley came to the UK from Africa as a young man in the 1990s, hoping but unable to continue working as a journalist. Instead he had to combine low-paid manual work, and journalism training at college, while caring for his young family. It was a stressful existence and he experienced a mental breakdown in 1997.

Stanley: And yeah. I was then diagnosed with bipolar disorder, and for the next four, five years, not even … 1997, 1998, yeah, about seven, eight years, next eight years I went through the revolving door cycle of going in and out of mental health, I was never mentally stable throughout that period. If I wasn't manic I would be at home, very, very severely depressed. Wasn't doing much, my life was not going anywhere.

And were you still working?

S: No. I couldn't work anymore. Dropped out of college, wasn't entitled to benefits because of my immigration status at the time. So, because I had a family and a young child, you know, we were being supported by social services, which was really difficult. They didn't give us any money, they gave us food vouchers, they paid our rent and that was about it. So, it was a very tough time then with my mental health. But it was in 2004 I had an admission, towards the back end of 2004.

But before that, even before that, throughout the eight years, you know, I had a fractured relationship with mental health professionals. I didn't trust them, I felt they didn't understand me and there was one important factor that they never did take into consideration, which was how important work was to me. You know, I remember the first consultant after my admission in 1997, I'd been discharged and was having an outpatient appointment with the consultant. And we were talking about, well, where do we go from here? And I said to him, well, I'd like to get on with my life, get on with my career, get back to journalism, get back to work. And his response was, forget journalism, it's too stressful a career for someone with your condition, you know.

And then a social worker, around about the same time, a few days later, my social worker – care coordinators as they're called now – well, my social worker, we had a similar conversation. And he actually told me, forget about work, consider yourself retired, enjoy the benefits you'll get for … the money, the free money you'll get for …

Consider yourself retired?

S: Consider yourself retired.

What age were you?

S: Twenty-nine. You know, so that didn't help.

Stanley goes on to describe one of his consultants.

S: You know, things weren't great between me and mental health services. I didn't trust them, I didn't have a great experience with them and I didn't have a great experience of my consultant at the time. You know, he was very distant, he never called me by my first name. It was always very formal. He didn't know my wife's name, he didn't know my children's names, it was as if all that was unimportant. It was all about medication, medication, medication.

I would go in for review meetings and it was so impersonal, I always got asked the same set of questions, textbook, from a textbook, I thought, you know. Can't remember exactly the questions, but I remember one question in particular that I always got asked, you know, he never asked, how are you, what's going on for you? You know, it was set questions, .one of the questions was, do you think you're special, do you think you've got superpowers?

And I knew what the questions were and I knew how to answer them, you know, if I said, yes, I have special powers, yes I think I'm special, I'd automatically be sectioned. So, one time, just after having answered the same question repeatedly, he asked me, do you think you're special? And I said, yes, of course I'm special. And he sat up, leaned forward in his chair, picked up his pen and, why are you special? I said, because I'm the son of a king. He says, oh, you're the son of a king. Yes of course, aren't we all children of God. You know, and that was just my way of being sarcastic and trying to show that your questions are stupid, insignificant, they're not helpful to me, they don't … it's not about me, it's not saying anything about me.

Later, Stanley used his knowledge of the system to get access to a different consultant.

S: But then, I managed … I used a loophole in the system to actually change my consultant psychiatrist. Because at each locality … because psychiatrists are allocated according to your catchment area, so each catchment was allocated two consultants. But they worked according … based on whichever GP surgery you were registered with determined which consultant psychiatrist you worked with.

So, I utilised that loophole and I switched GP services so I could switch to the other psychiatrist. Who, I heard, had a very good reputation; she was very understanding, she was very compassionate. And I just thought, she's got to be better than him, you know. So, I used that loophole, changed my consultant and my life changed.

You know, I remember my first meeting with my new consultant, it was at a time when I was struggling with my mental health, you know, I was becoming quite manic at the time. And she said to me ... we had a long discussion; with my previous consultant it was strictly fifteen minutes, that's it, fifteen minutes and no longer, and that was it.

With my new consultant, she sat and spoke to me for over an hour, and not even spoke, she listened to me. For over an hour she listened to me, asked me about, you know, who I am, what was important to me, asked about my wife, my children. She just wanted to let me speak about me, what was important to me, what mattered to me, you know.

And at the end of that hour, you know, she said to me, I can't cure your illness because there's no cure for bipolar disorder, as things stand. But, what we can do, and the important thing is, she said what we can do, is together, we can learn to manage your illness. And once we've learned to manage it, there is no reason why you cannot get on with your life, including getting back to work. And that was like a breath of fresh air for me.

So, when I met this new consultant, she actually put me in hospital that day. She said, I'm going to admit you today because, you know, we need to get on top of your mental health. But that was my last admission for the next ten years. For the next ten years I didn't have a single admission. I was back in work, I remained in work and my mental health was relatively stable. I had ups and down, blips, but because we had learned to manage it, we learned coping strategies, we learned how to recognise the early warning signs. But, I think the main thing for me was that I felt in control of my own life, of my own mental health. That was the biggest thing for me. And, of course, getting back into work was a big thing for me that helped me maintain my mental health.

And if you could just tell me a little bit more about, what are the things that she did that worked for you?

S: The main thing, the main thing that worked for me, was that she listened to me, and she saw me, the person, the husband, the father, the son. You know, previously, they saw the mentally ill patient, I was just a mentally ill patient, I was not a person. So previously, they saw the diagnosis rather than the person behind the diagnosis. So, that was the main thing for me, that she saw the person behind the diagnosis, she listened to me, she understood me and she gave me hope.

And that was the biggest difference. And I learned to trust, because in a patient–doctor relationship, if there is no trust then I'm not going to share with you when I'm not feeling great. In fear, because previously, if I just said, I don't feel great, it was straight to hospital. That was straight to hospital or an increase in medication, or a change in medication. Those seemed to be the only answers they had previously: it was, well, if you're feeling a bit depressed, we'll up your antidepressants. If you're feeling a bit manic, we'll up your anti-psychotics.

And if you're feeling a bit special, we'll section you.

S: Exactly. Now, where, with my new consultant, where she asked me about me, she asked me about my family, my interests, you know. What do I like doing, what do I do, and I learned to trust her. So, when I learned to trust her, I could answer honestly about how I'm feeling, knowing that, for her, putting me in hospital and even adjusting my medication was the last resort. She looked at other ways of dealing, like, if at the time my marriage was on the rocks and I was, you know, constantly rowing with my wife. And she saw that, and she said, well, increasing your medication is not going to stop you rowing with your wife, you know. So, she would look at other ways of how ... managing that situation, the reality. She looked at the reality and that, okay, this is what's causing you the stress, let's look at how we can deal with that situation, you know.

Story 18: Alan

Alan is a middle-aged man who once worked as a professional photographer. He was diagnosed as bipolar in the mid-1990s. He moved to Canada in 2000, returning to England in 2013 after the death of his father. Mental ill health was a feature of his life through these years, and shortly after his return to England he was admitted to hospital. He is very positive about the psychologist who subsequently cared for him.

Alan: I saw a psychologist and I was really lucky, because I was with her for just shy of two years. One of the reasons for that, she put it to me once: she does her own schedule, and I know it's six months or something, but two years? Absolutely amazing. We became really, really close, it was a really good relationship. The only reason why that ended, was because she went to another job.

She was the psychologist on the ward. On a personal level – psychology, it's all on a personal level – there was a really good relationship between us, I felt I could relax and talk with her.

And I would say to her as well, the times when I don't want to come down here, they're the times I need to come down here. So, there was a really kind of good understanding there. Well, she was really good at her job, and she taught me some really good, I found, CBT techniques. And also, they were one of the places that tried this out, and it was CFT, compassionate-focussed therapy.

Ah, I've not heard that one before.

A: Yeah, it was again treating the self with compassion, and one has just sprung to my mind now, imagining there's like a fog, and it's warm, and what colours are there, and you're walking into it. Things like that. Visualisation techniques. So being open to that as well, especially being, well, with my condition, also being "arty", creative, that had a real impact on me. So, yeah, that was like six, seven weeks, eight weeks. I'm not sure what happened in the end with it, but that was kind of a trial of it to see. I suppose the nature of the relationship was, after a while, being able to let go and make myself vulnerable, for so long, and also with her, it's kind of this mask, and I got so, so used to it, I can slip into it really quickly, but she was really good at picking up on that.

"How are you doing?" Yeah, I'm doing great, yeah. "But how are you really doing?" She was really, really good at that. Based on her … I can't think of the word …

Insight, perceptiveness?

A: Yeah, insight, perceptiveness, and also us actually having a really good bond as well. And also – a little thing, but there's no way you can prescribe any of this – but I'd see her on a Thursday, when one of my sessions was, and on the Fridays, I used to live near the hospital. So we would bump into each other, sit outside having a coffee, have a quick little chat, a hug, and then she'd go off. So, I kind of had that as well. So, we kind of had this, with hindsight anyway, this slightly unusual therapeutic relationship.

She was sort of setting aside the normal professional distance, and just behaving in a human way, it sounds?

A: Yeah, and it still felt like it was, it didn't feel, not inhuman, it didn't feel unhuman, but there was that additional little bit of an element, just like, how are you doing? Yeah, I'm doing … and you would anybody, any friend or whatever.

So, yeah, that definitely helped again for me. One of the biggest things she said for me, was me not appreciating what I can actually do. I haven't thought about this for a long while. One of the things was, if I can do something, because I can do it, anybody can. Well, I've realised that's not true. But that, for a long time, and she would really drill into that as well. She's really good at picking the points, she's very, very good at that, and that was some of the first ones, and I think, stop being humble, this is not a good thing, when it's put in with everything else. You're just downgrading, almost, yourself.

So, that was really, really good, to help me work with all that stuff. So now, when I'm now doing stuff, it has a lot more of an impact in the way people apparently talk about me, but I can actually be humble about that. It's, oh, that's great. 'Cause I know, oh I have those skills. It doesn't mean I …

Yes, so she was helping you value yourself at the kind of correct level?

A: Yeah, exactly, and then with that, then doing other things, it's like, oh my God, I can do that. It doesn't make me the bee's knees, it just means, that's great, I can do that, people like it. Oh, that's great, I'm really humbled by that.

So, yeah, she was amazing. So I think it was a combination of absolutely being top of her game, and also, I suppose, knowing as well, for me, that kind of certain boundaries weren't actually being adhered to. I think that kind of helped me think, well, relax, it's a bit unusual, it's what we make of it, rather than this is the prescribed therapeutic relationship. Like seeing her the day after, and you know, hi, a quick hug, have a good day?

So, I think for me it helped. I wouldn't say it became less clinical, less formal, should we say, and so, yeah, I think that's one of the reasons. And I'm sure, for two years, I mean, she did say to me towards the end, that she got a lot out of the sessions as well. And when she had her sessions, the psychologist, she would often talk about our sessions, and why it was so difficult for her to end the sessions. I think in the end her psychologist said, don't worry about it, you do your own schedule, it's up to you.

So, there was a really interesting relationship going on there. So, at the end of it all I gave her one of my abstract nature photographs, signed on the back, thank you. I gave her a hug, and she was crying. It was so sweet.

So, it's interesting, 'cause it sounds, I mean, the thing about a service user–health professional relationship, it often is kind of a one-way thing isn't it? Whereas, what you're describing is more of a two-way, it was more reciprocal?

A: Yeah, for sure.

And that in itself sounds like a therapeutic thing.

A: Yeah. She is, I'd say even better at her job, I'd say, rather than very good, she's very, very, very good, because she obviously realised that that's okay, and this would really, really help the work that we do. And there won't be any negative impact by pushing that boundary a bit. I hadn't thought about that before, actually. She knew, it didn't just happen. She would have thought about it, at least afterwards, when these things started to happen, and nip it in the bud, or no, that's okay, that actually …

So, it's like she knew where the boundaries were, but she made a judgement about where she could push them a bit?

A: Yeah absolutely. But I don't know how you could formulate that into suggestions, and how to work. You don't always have to keep to the boundaries. Well, I suppose so. But, that was the impact that it had. I think the important thing is that sometimes you need to tailor the therapy to the person that you're with.

The trust where Alan was treated has a forward-looking approach to engaging patients. He describes the transformative effect that his involvement in its "people participation" activities had on his mental well-being.

A: Really, really nervous, and really shy, but just slow, and the support, I mean it's a great team, and slowly doing different things. And I did talks at academic conferences, and NHS conferences and stuff, and to students, whatever. But, I always say to them, kind of before I started getting involved in this, I'd find it really difficult to talk amongst three people, and now I'm standing in front of 200.

So, first it was client contribution in the world, to the academic literature. But, yeah, for me it really did change everything, and I've spoken at the House of Lords and stuff, which I would never have imagined doing before. When I did my degree, four years as a student, somehow I managed to get away with only ever giving one seminar. But that was the nerves and the social anxiety, and that was why. Looking back with hindsight, it would be completely different now. But, that was kind of the – I can't think of the right word – not the baggage, but that's part of me, anyway.

So, yeah, loads of other different experiences along the way, but that's kind of my, I've now been involved for probably just shy of two years.

So, the way you're describing it, it seems as though becoming involved in the participation work is absolutely relevant to your recovery?

A: Oh, absolutely.

Very interesting. And tell me a bit about that, so you've said something about giving talks and things, tell me about the range of activities that you do.

A: For me, anyway, doing workshops with DLR [Docklands Light Railway] staff, London Transport, 'cause they encounter, obviously, people that might be in crisis, so it's sharing my own journey with them, and also being quite open about my condition. So, I'm happy to talk about it. I always say to them at the end, 'cause they're big, burly East End guys, most of them, asking for help isn't a weakness, it's a sign of strength. So I try and get that across to them.

Business students, business apprentices in Canary Wharf. Get the younger generation, and they pass it on to their friends. So, I do that. Training researchers now, or service users to become researchers. Been to Manchester, Birmingham and Belfast, to talk about people participation, what it is, the impact that it's had on me, the research project, and how beneficial it can be for a trust as well, because who knows the best about the services that are provided? The people that receive them. In saying that to trainee nurses, you can see them, oh yeah. It's like, seriously, that's never crossed your mind before? But, for whatever reason it hasn't, so it's like, okay, I can do this and I get really nervous, but I can actually talk in front, and hopefully inspire some people.

And it's actually providing many of the things that other people would get from paid employment, like validation and responsibility?

A: Yeah, and it's helped me, kind of – it sounds really strange when I say it out loud – find my place in the world. And it's reminded me sometimes of skills and talents, I forgot I had, as well as learning new ones. 'Cause, yeah, everybody up here would not recognise me, if it was three years ago, and I walked in. They wouldn't. So, I can see the impact that's had. And it also, being able to make a contribution that's valued, into the services, as well. And it's like, I suppose, I'm not a service user union rep, I can't speak for all service users, but being able to have that voice and directly affect change, and having it valued, and it's not lip service.

It's very empowering then, so that you can make a difference, which is a difference worth having.

A: Yeah, absolutely, yeah, it's really, really empowering. It never crossed my mind until it was pointed out to me at the hospital, the lead nurse – I've gone over there and sat on interview panels with him – kind of said to me, so we've never said this before, this rarely happens. I goes, what rarely happens? Well, you were on the ward for a long, long time. Yeah. We rarely, if ever, get to see somebody the other side. They said, it doesn't happen. And they said, so it's so great to see you, and now doing all that stuff, and hearing about all the stuff you do. It's great, 'cause from there how you were back then, to how you are now.

A lot of the time they've no idea what happens to the people who pass through?

A: You only see them in crisis, you only see them on the ward, you've got no idea what happens to their life afterwards.

Story 19: Nathan

Nathan started having treatment for mental health problems at around the age of 11 after his school became concerned about his hyperactive behaviour. When he spoke to us he was 17. Nathan, who identifies as gay, has had problems with his family and with his schools. He contrasts the problems he encountered at school, with his positive experiences of the Child and Adult Mental Health Service (CAMHS), especially the relief of being believed and supported.

Nathan: Essentially, it was really difficult in high school because not only are you juggling sexuality, you're also juggling that I wasn't the best in maths and English because of bullying because of other stuff I was focussing on obviously, so I have changed schools. But because of that it was so difficult, I remember the amount of times that I just didn't want to be here and I was so suicidal and CAMHS, luckily, they do believe you if you say that. So if you say, I'm not in a good place, they will work with your school to make sure that you're not doing anything bad.

I remember someone I was seeing because they knew that I had a massive fear of certain subjects because I just got bullied in them; they made a plan with the school that I would only do half days. But that in itself was a really big thing for a therapist to get involved with the school and basically move your whole schedule just so you don't get bullied. That wasn't until the end of year eight, so you can imagine how the first two years were, they weren't the best.

I remember the teachers would just assume that everything you were doing was attention seeking or it was because of a bad family member or it would be because, oh, it runs in the family or you're just dumb. They wouldn't … I remember I tried telling one of my teachers that my dad wasn't the best person and they just wouldn't believe me, they spoke to him once and went, oh, no, he's fine, and didn't believe me and didn't report it to a social worker or anything like that.

So you can imagine how that worked, the first person you're meant to trust is a teacher, so you can imagine it wasn't the best two-year period, but the second you come to CAMHS it's completely different, they believed me instantly, they offered to speak to you on the phone.

So I just went in, within my first few sessions I said, look, this is what my home life is like, I'm not saying this because I want attention or anything, I'm just telling you because I told my school, they didn't believe me.

And within the next few days we were having a meeting and they were saying how the school wasn't being professional because I was saying that I was being abused by my dad, not only that I was being bullied in school, the teacher didn't believe me in that. They were also saying that I was struggling with certain subjects and they, again, didn't believe me on that and I was saying I didn't have many friends and they didn't believe me.

I was saying that I didn't feel safe leaving school and going home. I was really anxious and a bit scared because my dad would stalk me when I came outside school and threaten me and whatnot. And the school didn't believe me about that either but, luckily, CAMHS, they did believe me and trust me and take me seriously. Because what they used to do is some of the therapists would wait outside with me until the taxi arrives, until my mum arrived. And I just thought that's such a small thing but such a big thing at the same time and it can really go a long way to make someone feel comfortable and safe.

Nathan describes the importance of the therapist establishing a good rapport with him:

N: I remember when I first came here the only reason I was able to open up was because the therapist I was seeing was able to tone it down and be a bit more funny with me, a bit laid back, and so I trusted him more. And that was a great technique to do to a 13-year-old. But had it been someone very serious who couldn't do that, I wouldn't have opened up, I probably would have turned my back on CAMHS and thought, well, I've already seen someone, I'm not going to bother with any more. So I think that's a really important quality: to able to adjust to your audience or client, depending on the situation.

He also explains the importance of continuity of care.

N: I was seeing this very nice lady for kind of a longish period of time; they offered me, I think, sixteen sessions or something. After the sixteen sessions obviously I was fine and I stopped seeing them for a couple of months but when I had a bit of an issue, so I came back and I said I would like to see someone again, the doctor referred me. And because I'd already seen this person they asked her if she'd be able to see me again so I didn't have to go through it again. And I think, again, she was able to see me which was really good.

So now I'm seeing the same person that I was seeing last time, so I didn't have to waste two or three weeks going through everything again.

Yes, as far as you're concerned, you'd much rather see somebody that you already know than start again from scratch?

N: Yeah, well, it's mainly because here they don't mean to but they have a problem where if you say something, when they put it on the file the next person who looks at it will somehow get it wrong. Whether it'll be they've read it wrong or they've misinterpreted it, and they don't mean it in a rude way but they say, oh, yeah, you did something. No, no, I didn't … and then you have a week or two weeks correcting them and it's obviously annoying, especially when you've seen someone for five years there's a lot of stuff to correct.

Nathan's experiences of CAMHS services have varied. He describes one unfortunate incident.

N: I had one person who on my first session they tried to diagnose me with something without speaking to me; within the first three lines they went, oh, you're autistic. I'm not autistic, I've done the test multiple times, I'm not. And you could imagine how that would be after seeing someone for two years and they have to leave and then you see this new person you've been waiting months for, months longer than they said you would be waiting, and within the first session like, oh, yeah, you're autistic, we don't need to see each other anymore. Yeah, you can imagine how that was.

We have a broader discussion about labels and diagnoses.

N: So the problem CAMHS does have is it doesn't like labels that much, which is understandable because a lot of people react negatively to labels, but labels can be really good because if you're having an issue and you're suffering a symptom of something, you know what to Google, but you know not to Google issues with breathing if you're having a panic attack because you might think you're having a heart attack or something and you rush to the hospital and nothing's wrong with you, you're having a panic attack or something like that.

So I think it depends on the person. I'm not someone who'd believe the first thing I see on Google so I think it's quite helpful for me to look things up. But, that being said, I had a friend of mine who'd believe everything she reads online and so it would be horrible and terrible for her to Google something to try and understand it more because she'd be completely wrong.

Yeah, it's interesting, it's a delicate balancing act then, isn't it, between the labelling that gives you some understanding of the symptoms and what to do, versus the sense of being labelled by other people and, therefore, not being treated as a person, just a set of conditions?

N: So because I'm very open about it, I don't care about the stigma, so because of that I think I'm able to look at the labels as a different approach to some people. So I'm able to look at it and see, well, it's not that they're defining me but, in fact, they're just defining how I can get help.

So for me I always see a label as kind of like a describing word in a way, I can use it in the sense of if I'm having an issue I can say, oh, I'm just OCD, not, I'm suffering with OCD, I could just say, well, I'm having a bit of an OCD epidemic right now.

Yes, because for you, you can take an analytical approach and it just helps to make sense. So have you collected quite a lot of labels over the years?

N: Yeah.

And is that in itself problematic?

N: Oh, definitely, it can be really problematic for some people. So with me it's not but, as I said, that's just because I'm the type of person I am.

But other people – it can be a terrible thing to diagnose them with something because then they think there's something wrong with them, so I think it depends on the approach and the person and the relationship the client and the therapist has.

What you're saying is actually this is quite a difficult area where the therapists need to be quite skilled and where the opportunity for misunderstandings is probably quite big?

N: Yeah, so many people have an issue where they get diagnosed with something and they get really upset because they've misunderstood it. So I think the best approach probably would be to look at the relationship the therapist and the client has, if they've got a good connection, then they could diagnose them with something and label it and know there's not going to be a miscommunication there, which is positive.

But obviously, if you've been seeing someone for a short amount of time it's probably not the best idea to label them immediately because they're going to then feel like, well, what do you know, you've only seen me for four weeks or something? Even if it's really obvious.

So I think the approach would be to speak to the parents because obviously parents play a massive part in mental health. Because otherwise the problem is when you tell the child, I think you might have something, they hear, I have something. So they can't see that you're saying, "might", not, "have", so they will go, well, I've definitely got this one thing, so they go and tell everyone at school, they tell the teachers and they don't have it and then they're really embarrassed and they get bullied for it.

Yes, it's a minefield, isn't it, is what you're saying?

N: Yeah.

On another occasion an initial misdiagnosis was an opportunity for a therapist to listen and to admit that they were wrong.

N: So my issue was when I thought I had OCD, and I do, but they thought I didn't have it for so long, so when I finally told this newer person, they said, well, I don't think you have it but we'll do the test and if you get sixteen out of twenty we'll do the test or whatever – I can't remember exactly because it was so long ago. But I did get pretty high in that test and she was like, oh, I was wrong, okay, well, that's good.

So because she was able to put her own feelings aside it turned out I did get diagnosed with something that I do have and they thought I didn't.

Yes, I quite like the fact that she said, I was wrong, and she was able to admit that without it being a big deal.

N: Yeah, yeah, it's really good to be able to admit, okay, even with all my training I was wrong, it's really helpful. You can imagine how it would be if you're continuously asking them to give you the bit of paper so you could fill it in and they tell you for years you don't have it and you finally do, and it's so good to hear them say, okay, I was wrong.

It's so helpful when they're able to say, I was wrong, and ignore their training for a slight moment or so. Because you get some people where they go, well, I'm trained in this area so I understand it maybe a bit more than you might. And it's like, yeah, but everyone is different, so you might end up having something, they just might not be able to notice it.

Because obviously, as much as you should be open in therapy, you're never going to be yourself truly, there's always going to be some things that you don't bring. Whether that's because of the anxiety of it or you just don't ever think to mention it, but there are always some things that you don't mention and that's why it's really important to listen to the person and just do the test, if it is a test, whatever you want to get diagnosed for. But if there's a test it's really important to do it, because there are some cases where they find out stuff they didn't know about you because you never thought to mention it and it turns out that that small thing helps you so much in getting diagnosed and it can really affect you.

The interview with Nathan concludes with a story touching on the themes of trust, honesty and openness.

N: If the client doesn't think you're polite or nice, they're not going to bother with you or they're going to lie to you. Because a big issue I had when I started seeing my second therapist, I found myself lying to make myself sound better than I was so they would let me leave the trust because I just didn't like the person I was seeing. But, luckily, I ended up just having confidence and just going to reception and saying, look, I need to see someone else, I do not like this person at all.

And they were really nice to me about it and they put me on the waiting list to see someone else. But if I didn't have that, I could have then gone home and done something really stupid because I didn't like the person I was seeing.

It's a really interesting set of circumstances because in a way you were in quite a dangerous position because you were not telling the truth to your therapist, you didn't like the therapist, and you did quite a brave thing by saying, actually this is not working for me.

N: Yeah, especially because I know that I had a big fear that the reception would tell them that: he said he didn't like you. And I would be told, no, you can't see someone else because this is person you're assigned to. But, luckily, I got over that fear and asked; they don't do that, they, luckily, don't do that at all but obviously that can be such a big fear for some people.

So I think if the therapist thinks you're hiding something it's good when they say that, I think you're hiding something. Or at least in my case I like people being direct with me. So one thing my therapist did do which I found really helpful: on the first session they get you to write a list of triggers and a list of things that you like or they just ask you and they write it down. So because of that she will always know to be direct with me so I don't feel like I'm being ... I don't feel like I'm just being treated as an idiot.

So because of that in sessions she'll be very direct and very blunt, which works for me and that's how we have a very strong connection, I'm able to open up about things because she took the time to ask me what I like, what I think is good, what I think helps me.

And that, again, is such a small thing that not many people think of doing but that's such a good thing to do because it can really open up the client to actually want to talk about themselves a bit more, to talk about what bothers them and what doesn't, to talk about how you like speaking to them and things like that.

Oh, you describe it as a little thing but I would say it is actually fairly funda-mental, understanding what matters to the client.

N: Yeah, I think the reason some people don't ask is because they think they can probably just assume. But I think it is so helpful when they do ask and it's something that I haven't seen much of and I really hope to see more of it because that small thing this one person did made me want to go back and see the same person again when I was feeling depressed. Otherwise I could have been self-harming and then done something stupid at the end.

So that one thing opening up so many opportunities where I was able to save myself from something really stupid. And I think that's why it's so important they do something like that and that's why I really hope that I see more of it.

Story 20: Lucy

Lucy is a retired consultant psychiatrist who has suffered from mental ill health all her life from teenagehood onwards. She describes how as a healthcare professional she knows her way around the system but even so it hasn't always been easy to find the right care. Lucy also tells of her experience when she was hospitalised with sepsis in Chapter 5 (Story 14).

To start with, can you tell me, what is mood disorder?

Lucy: Mood disorder is a type of mental illness. It's depression. Anxiety is sometimes put in with the mood disorders, but it's depression, mania, it's disorders of a change of mood, so where your mood can go from anything from high to low, to things in between, or a mixture of the two in some cases.

I'd like to mainly focus on one aspect, which is how, over the years, you've managed to find your way around the system to get the care that you need. But I guess before we do that, it would be helpful just to have a rehearsal or a summary of who you are, what your job has been, and when you first realised you were ill.

L: Sure. Yes, I'm a retired consultant psychiatrist and I first realised that I had problems with my mental health when I was a medical student, although, looking back, it's clear that I had quite severe anxiety as a teenager as well. And I saw a psychiatrist for the first time when I was a medical student, and then I've had quite a lot of psychotherapy, and I've also been on medication pretty much … well, I think continuously, but not on the same type, since 1995, or 1994, so a long time. And I've been under the care of psychiatrists, which probably would not have happened had I not been a psychiatrist, I have to say, although it might have done at times. But I've had pretty much continuous care, apart from a period in the late 1990s when I was reasonably well for a while, and then I was out of contact, but since the late 1990s to the present, I've been under the care of a psychiatrist. And I think I've been very fortunate in that, and I can't imagine how a GP would have managed my illness, but I know there are lots of people like me who would have only seen a GP, so I think I've been very lucky.

And tell me why it's because you're a psychiatrist that you got to see a psychiatrist, and what difference does seeing a psychiatrist make for the kind of illness that you have?

L: I really negotiated my treatment myself, which I think would be really hard now because everything is so intensely bureaucratic. I was working at a time when it was possible for, say … without anybody saying, oh, sorry, we've not got a contract with them. And I know that doesn't happen now because I've met people who have said, I desperately need help but I've been told I have to come to the service, and I work in it and I'm not prepared to come here. And that's changed just recently for doctors, in that doctors can now be referred nationally to the service that Clare Gerada set up, the Mental Health Service for Doctors, but that's only the last month or so.

And I think, as a psychiatrist, I was aware that many of my colleagues were not people I would want to see… I hate to say this but … When I've taught specialist registrars, and they've said, oh, GPs are dreadful. And I said, well, there's a lot of variety amongst GPs and some of them are very good, some of them are not that interested in psychiatry. I said, how many of your colleagues would you be willing to see as a patient? And then they all laugh, because everybody knows exactly what I mean. But there's this kind of stupid delusion that somehow everybody gets the same care, and they don't, and there's no choice. And I just knew that I wanted to see someone who could offer me more of a kind of psychodynamic perspective, as well as a psychological perspective, so I actually arranged to see one of my colleagues, and he/she was willing to see me, in the 1990s.

Prior to that, I'd seen a psychotherapist who was also arranged via a colleague. All that was done through kind of colleagues' networks … It became more formalised because I was then seen by the specialist affective disorders people, and that was good because I think, at that time, things were a bit more complicated.

For you?

L: For me, in terms of my illness, but I think I probably could have been discharged from there now, but I'm still under their follow-up. And I know, had I been a patient, I would have been discharged years ago, an ordinary patient.

What, because you weren't ill enough?

L: They just don't provide long-term follow-up for people with severe … with my kind of illness, who are not local to them. You know, there are very few specialist mood disorder centres. Depression that's not psychotic is assumed to be within the realms of outpatient and GP care. A lot of GPs are struggling with people that they shouldn't be struggling with. IAPT [Improving Access to Psychological Therapies] services very often won't see them, because when suicide is mentioned, people don't get seen. There are a large number of people who are kind of stuck between primary and secondary care, and they get seen and then they get discharged back to the GP, and often they're left on medication, which they shouldn't be left on. And I used to see them in XXX, because I was working in a primary care service, and I would see people that really should have been having longer-term follow-up. So, I mean, I was on lithium for quite some time, for depression. I've known people discharged back to the GP who were on lithium for depression, and with no kind of indication of how long they should stay on it, because no one knows. And until fairly recently, and in many places it's still the case, it's just GPs are very angry about it, you'd have to refer back through the system again, to get people seen again, or wait until they're in crisis. So I've still had follow-up from XXX, and that's been great, although the service came close to being cut about two years ago, but then they gave it a reprieve, and that would have meant there wouldn't have been a specialist service, and if I wanted to see a psychiatrist, I probably would have gone privately.

So can you just tell me a little bit more about the illness that you suffer from? You call it … is it a specialist affective disorder?

L: Well, it's a specialist affective disorders unit that I go to, but that's a special unit for people who have mood disorders. In other words, it's not just ordinary general psychiatry, it's a disorder that specialises in people with mood disorders, so they have a lot of concentrated expertise, especially around medication, that the average general psychiatrist possibly wouldn't know all of the latest evidence, wouldn't know the research. They used to have a psychologist attached to them as well, and that's been cut, but it used to be a unit that you could go to if you weren't getting better otherwise. In the US, there are specialist depression centres pretty much around the country, because there's a recognition that mood disorders are complex and sometimes people are left on medication, or don't recover when they could be much better. And they also look after people with bipolar disorder as well, so it's the whole range of mood problems.

And are you saying that really you've only been able to access this treatment because you're on the inside and you're in the know?

L: I think so. And I see young people now in medicine and who can't do that because it's not so easy to get that route because everything is so bureaucratic. So I have somehow managed to be under the care of XXX trust, despite living here for a very long time … Under the radar, exactly how it was when I was in training, when my consultant looked after a number of people, and when he went on holiday, when I was a senior registrar, he would say, I'm a bit worried about x, y and z. He's a consultant, she's a consultant, if anything goes wrong, you know, this is what to do. And there was a kind of recognition that we did take care of people who worked within the system.

So if you were a member of the public and not a doctor, what would your kind of journey have looked like? How different would your journey have been?

L: It would have largely stayed with the GP, with possible long-term outpatient clinic appointments where I'd see different junior doctors who would tinker with my medication.

That's what it would have been like?

L: Yeah, and now I would almost certainly have been discharged back to a GP.

And in terms of your state of health, what difference would that have made?

L: I think I would not have been able to stay at work and I may well have come off my medication ... I certainly reached a point at various times when it was no longer helpful and it had to be changed, until I found the right one. And my current consultant has said that he thinks that if I hadn't stayed on it, I would have ended up in hospital. He says it's the fact that I have been very persistent with my treatment that has kept me out of hospital. I think I would have been in hospital at some point in my life, but I've managed to avoid it.

Have you never been an inpatient?

L: No ... When I was a medical student, a doctor I saw wanted to admit me and I wouldn't have it, and I've resisted ever since, and I never needed it ... I've had long periods off work, but certainly my current doc says he thinks I would have been a lot worse if I'd have not stayed on the medication, and I think he's absolutely right, I think I would have ended up an inpatient. I've been very persistent with trying to ensure that I stayed with treatment, and with the best treatment.

And that's because you know about what the options are.

L: I know, yeah.

So why do you think it is that in mental health there is this lack of choice about where you go that is different from physical health? There are all these kind of boundaries, you know, you have to go and seek mental health from a certain area, whereas if you've got a physical problem, you've got patient choice and Choose and Book.

L: Well, in the 1980s, when I was a junior doctor, we saw a lot of people from outside of the area. There was quite a lot of choice. In fact, I remember someone saying something like a third of our admissions were outside area, because we had people like X, who was an expert in his field and would see people with complex grief problems, from all over the XXX of England. And then, when managerialism came in in a very strong way, and at the same time, there was a retrenching of the mental health service, to say we are looking after only the most severely mentally ill, and that is community orientated, and you have to be cared for by a team, and a team covers a patch, and so we went through fairly rigid sectorisation. And then it became impossible to see someone from outside your sector, never mind outside your area, so if you didn't get on with your sector doctor, well, then you'd had it, really.

And I remember in XXX, we were able and willing to see people from the other sectors, but some of the consultants were not, and they were very rigid about it. And the GPs loathed it because sometimes they had patients across different sectors, and they loathed the fact that sometimes half their patients got a better service to the other half, and I fought very much to try and get us to be attached to GPs, not to sectors, so that we could work with GPs. But again, that did mean that ... It kind of ignored the fact there was considerable variation in quality ...

It varied in quality among the general practice or ... ?

L: No, amongst the psychiatrists.

Tell me a bit more about that.

L: Well, it's always been a shortage speciality ... If you get a good reputation as a centre, then you can fill your consultant posts, but if you get a bad reputation, then you end up it just being a string of locums. And I've watched different trusts go up and down in that over the time I've been a consultant. I mean, there was a period when XXX had a really good reputation, so it had all of its posts filled, and then there was a period when it went downhill and they couldn't keep staff. YYY went terribly downhill for the same reason, because it was chaotic, and I had a couple of trainees ... who went off to work in ZZZ, lasted three months, and said, well, if I stay here, I'm going to turn into the sort of consultant I don't want to be, so they moved. And then that means that that area just goes completely downhill and you end up with a series of locums, and it's pretty awful, because some of the locums are people who are okay, but some of them are dreadful.

And to what extent do you think are the public in the dark about this?

L: I think the public know about it if they've got relatives who have got mental health problems, and they also imagine that if they go privately, it will be fine, whereas they don't realise that most of the people working in the system are the people who also do private work, so they're not actually necessarily getting better quality by going privately. You've still got to know who the consultants are if you go privately. You know, I will not go and see anybody; I would only go and see people who I know, from talking to others, are worth seeing ... I don't want anybody insisting on tinkering with my medication who doesn't know what they're doing, because it's been very finely balanced at times.

So in terms of finding your way, I guess one could say you are in a privileged position.

L: Yeah.

When it works and you find the right service for you, what does that feel like?

L: It feels safe. It feels like you've got someone who you know that you can phone up if you need to. You can go and see them earlier if you need to. You haven't got to go through … You haven't got to go and argue with somebody in order to be seen. For me, it's always been very important that someone has been prepared to talk to me about other things going on in my life, other than the fact that I need to just take the tablets … They might not be a psychotherapist but they've got knowledge of what therapy is about. And that I feel like they're up-to-date in what they are doing.

And I talk to service users on social media sometimes and they tell me things that are happening, and I know that they're not getting the most up-to-date treatment, necessarily … and I say, look, I can't give you advice, but I just say, my doctor has tried x, y and z and he is a specialist.

I do know that people who are not specialists in mood disorders are often reluctant to try things that there might be some evidence for. I got very, very ill about two years ago … and I had to go on a second antidepressant, so I was on two. And my doctor put me on something that's off-label, but it's used in the US, and he prescribed it. My GP didn't, but then my GP agreed to prescribe it. That would never have been tried by a general consultant, but it got me better.

That somebody who is up-to-date and reading the journals and all the rest of it.

L: Yeah, and doing the research

And when it's not been so good and you've struggled to find the right service for you, what does that feel like?

L: Well, I've been lucky. I would say that there's only been one doctor I've seen that I didn't feel able to talk to that easily, and that was the first person I saw after the consultant I saw for years retired, and I didn't find her quite so easy to talk to, but she was still there. It was just that we didn't feel that comfortable because we'd worked previously together, and she just wasn't really a person I felt that at ease with. And it's funny, because I've seen her at other occasions since I stopped seeing her, and she's so different when she meets me now. She was uncomfortable. But I've not been in that position, other than with GPs ... I had the same GP for twenty years, and then when he retired, it was quite hard, because I felt like there was no one who really understood my story, whereas my old GP had seen me through quite a long period of time when I'd been ill.

One of the things that I've discovered so far is that, when I listen to people's stories, general practice comes in for really quite a bad press, and this is not to do with mental illness, this is just in general. Really quite a lot of bad press. So when the GP service is good, from your point of view, what is it like?

L: When a GP service is good, you feel like there's somebody who's on your side, who will actually help you to get to where you need to be seen, and won't argue with what the specialist is saying, which is really important, because I've certainly known situations, when I was a consultant, where I would be prescribing something and the GP would be refusing to do it, saying, oh, we've had a letter through that we're not supposed to do this. And you'd say, well, actually that's not supposed to interfere with individual patient care decisions. I think we're very fortunate living up here. I say that because the local practice out here has no difficulty filling its posts. It's because, as you can imagine, GPs want to come and work out here, because it's nice. So I've always had good GPs, but the practice has got much bigger: there are a lot more people working part-time in it now, and there's more of a sense of it being not as easy to get to know doctors. For a long time, I saw a doctor who was a bit kind of unconventional in many ways, but I could talk to him, and he wasn't the least bit afraid of asking me difficult questions either. I mean, he was the person who put me on antidepressants to start off with. He was really good, but I do find that they're kind of more detached and business-like almost, now. It is more of a job for them and less of a vocation, I know that. But I'm getting to know a couple of them now that I find it easier to talk to, but there are twelve of them now, and there used to be five, and it's just not the same. But at least we don't have a shortage of GPs here and we don't have locums.

So now, thinking about your professional work, you will have seen/observed/ experienced people who have felt that they've found the service that's right for them. What difference does it make to them?

L: I think it helps people get better, I really do. I really feel strongly that what's happened within healthcare is that there has been – and I think this is particularly important for mental healthcare – is there's been a complete doing away with the importance of the relationship. And I see it in community mental health services and I see it when I talk to people who experience community mental health services. We're treating people as objects ... If you're suicidal, what keeps you alive is the relationship you have with the mental health professional. Having a different person come and see you each day and just say, do you feel like killing like yourself today? does not keep people alive. And I kept people alive through the power of my relationship with them, and by the fact that they grew to trust me, and I grew to trust them, and we worked on that and I was able to give them hope. If you don't know somebody, you can't give them hope, and if you don't know somebody, they will not trust you when you say you're going to get better. And all of that has gone. It's all become commodified. It's all about just getting people through the system. I think it's really affected risk in services, because I think risk has just become something that everyone's scared of. But I worked with some very complex people in my career.

When you see people, when they've struggled to find the right service for them, what impact does that have on them?

L: Well, they start to get really hopeless about it and they start to feel that services have got nothing to offer them and feel very cut off. I've met people on social media, through time on there, who have basically been told that services have got nothing to offer them, and they're discharged. You know, I just can't believe that, but that's what they do.

And why do you think the psychiatrist profession have allowed this commodification that you describe?

L: I think they've allowed it because they thought it would make their work easier, because they felt overburdened, but it's actually resulted in their work being less satisfactory ... A lot of that, I think, resulted in making it harder to recruit to the profession.

MENTAL HEALTH AND MENTAL ILLNESS: REFLECTIONS AND RESPONSES TO THESE STORIES

Immediate questions

1. What was the significance of work for Stanley? How might the NHS have acted differently in the light of this?

2. Stanley "used a loophole" to get the consultant he wanted. How do you feel about him "working the system" to get the care he needed? What issues does it raise?
3. Lucy also "worked the system", using her knowledge as a psychiatrist to get the care she needed. How do you feel about this? What issues does it raise?
4. Alan is very positive about his involvement in patient engagement activities. What are the benefits and risks of patients becoming involved in these ways? What is the role of the NHS in supporting such activities for service users?
5. How would you describe the pros and cons of labels and diagnoses, based on Nathan's experiences?

Strategic questions
1. What does good-quality mental healthcare look and feel like according to these testimonies?
2. What part can agencies play in combatting the structural discrimination that is often experienced by mental health service users such as Stanley and Nathan?
3. What might be the barriers to being able to focus on the person as well as the illness?
4. Why is the relationship between therapist and patient so important in these stories? What are the features of a good relationship? What is needed to create the conditions for good relationships? What obstacles need to be overcome?
5. What can individual mental health professionals and managers do to join up care better between specialist mental health services, primary care and other agencies, such as schools?
6. Why is continuity of care important? How can it be promoted?

REFERENCES

Bignall, T., S. Jeraj, E. Helsby and J. Butt (2019) *Racial Disparities in Mental Health: Literature and evidence review* (London: Race Equality Foundation), https://raceequalityfoundation.org.uk/wp-content/uploads/2020/03/mental-health-report-v5–2.pdf (accessed 5 January 2021).

Mental Health Foundation (2016) *Fundamental Facts about Mental Health 2016*, www.mentalhealth.org.uk/sites/default/files/fundamental-facts-about-mental-health-2016.pdf (accessed 5 January 2021).

NHS (2019) *NHS Mental Health Implementation Plan 2019/20–2023/4*, www.longtermplan.nhs.uk/wp-content/uploads/2019/07/nhs-mental-health-implementation-plan-2019-20-2023-24.pdf (accessed 5 January 2021).

NHS Digital (2018) "Mental health of children and young people in England 2017", official statistics, 19 November, https://digital.nhs.uk/data-and-information/publications/statistical/mental-health-of-children-and-young-people-in-england/2017/2017 (accessed 5 January 2021).

NHS England (2016) *The Five Year Forward View for Mental Health*, www.england.nhs.uk/publication/the-five-year-forward-view-for-mental-health (accessed 28 March 2021).

※ 7 ※

OLDER AGE AND
END OF LIFE

INTRODUCTION

As the charity Age UK points out, poor health in later life is not inevitable and is not irreversible (Age UK, 2019). We live in an era in which society is getting older, and healthy ageing is a policy goal and a call to action for many. Nevertheless, as a whole we are more reliant on health and care services as we age, more likely to receive a cancer diagnosis and more likely to live with long-term conditions. The majority of people over 85 are living with three or more conditions. Many older people live in loneliness and social isolation, which can harm their physical and mental well-being. COVID-19 has tragically highlighted the increased susceptibility of older people to certain infectious diseases.

The ways in which health and care services are organised do not always reflect the fact that older people are often the main users. As discussed in Chapter 4, the NHS tends to organise care reactively around single condition pathways, and is weaker at delivering proactive, person-centred care that coordinates different services around the patient. We have noted the importance, reflected in numerous policy documents and research reports, of joined-up care for patients throughout the course of life, particularly as services are provided by so many different health and care organisations, and with varying funding arrangements. At no stage is coordinated care more vital than in older age and at the end of life. This is not only because of the complexity of health and care arrangements, but also because many of the carers are also older and may be vulnerable themselves.

Older people are particularly affected by the under-provision of primary and community services, the underfunding of social care and patchy support for family carers. There is often poor coordination between NHS and social care – the problem of delayed discharge from hospital being the classic example. The NHS frequently struggles to respond to the needs of people with dementia (which features in a number of the stories in this chapter) and with frailty – both conditions which become more likely with age. Ageism is widely prevalent, according to the World Health Organization, which is harmful to the health of older people and can have an adverse effect on their access to services (WHO, 2015).

Scandals of poor care, for example at the Mid Staffordshire NHS Foundation Trust (Mid Staffordshire NHS Foundation Trust Public Inquiry, 2013), have highlighted failures to respect older people's basic dignity in hospital, and there are perennial concerns about the quality and sustainability of care in residential homes.

We have chosen to include stories about living with and looking after someone with dementia here rather than earlier as it is mainly – although not always – a disease of older age. Around 850,000 people in the UK live with dementia, including one in six people over the age of 80, with the number expected to increase to over 1 million by 2025 (NHS, 2020). Dementia is therefore becoming a critically important issue, in terms of the high personal and social costs related to the disease (Oliver, 2015).

Everyone should be able to expect services and support that work for them at the end of life, such as access to good palliative care and pain management, emotional and spiritual support, and respect for their personal choices and dignity. For many, hospice care is seen as the gold standard. It has been a policy goal in recent years to enable people to die in a place of their choosing, but the broader goal of enabling a "good death" remains a challenge for the NHS. In the UK, the Liverpool Care Pathway was seen by many as a humane and minimally invasive way of caring for people close to death, but for others it was viewed as the pathway to euthanasia, and it was scrapped (Nasim, 2014). The judgement about when to stop trying to save someone's life and start enabling them to die with dignity is not always straightforward.

THE STORIES

In Chapter 1 (Section 2, p. 4), we offer a description of patient-centred care, in general, as:

- Understanding and valuing what matters to patients
- Seeing the whole person

- Respecting people's rights and autonomy
- Being customer focussed

There are five stories in this chapter. **Robert** is in his 80s and has a heart condition and also stomach and joint problems. He became involved with patient participation in the NHS after retirement. **Rabiya** cares for her mum, who has dementia and doesn't speak English well. **James** (whom we have already met in Chapter 2, Story 2) looked after his mother for ten years after her diagnosis of dementia until she died. **Sheila** cares for her husband who has dementia and has battled to get a diagnosis and care in place. **Kauri**'s dad died recently of pancreatic cancer. She narrates many episodes of excellent care and support.

Story 21: Robert

Robert is in his 80s and has a heart condition and also stomach and joint problems. He became involved with patient participation in the NHS after retirement. He is concerned about fragmentation and communication problems in the NHS, as well as difficulties in getting an appointment with the GP, and he also notes a lack of clarity about the role of the district nurse. He describes good experiences of being treated in an NHS hospital as well as being an NHS patient in a private hospital.

Robert: You have to go back to, believe it or not, 1943, when I was foolish enough to put in my mouth a metal wheel, it had spokes in the middle, and it perforated my bowel, and I was in hospital for the better part of ten months then …

I've got a wound from that and it is bloated now. I have to go twice a week as a minimum to see a community nurse to have it dressed. And I see a consultant about the stomach wound. On one occasion the consultant said, can I see your wound? And I said, well, you will have to have a nurse to do the wound back again – so he didn't see it. He didn't bother. It would be the best part of … well, three hours, shall we say, driving there and driving back and waiting. Quite honestly, I think it's a waste of time going to see him. I think it can be done by phone just as easily.

And another thing: he said, if, in other circumstances – by that time I'd been diagnosed with a heart problem – if you didn't have the heart problem, we'd probably operate on it. Well, I'm not certain whether I want an operation because at the age of 83 or 82, or whatever I was at that time, I would have felt that, well, I don't particularly want to volunteer for a further operation at my age. I'm prepared to put up with this … I have had to vastly change my clothes because none will fit me; but he said, sorry, we will consider an operation now. But we didn't really discuss any more, I didn't want to, in fairness to him. But there should have been some liaison between him and the heart person. They're in their own silo doing their own thing.

So, with the knees and the hips, have they all been done in a private hospital, as an NHS patient?

R: No. The last operation that I had the second time here was at the local NHS hospital, and apart from not having a room on my own, one with my own television and everything else, the service was equally as good as it was at the private hospital.

I did feel that the physios there, they felt they've made it because they've got to a private hospital, and the service was more along the lines of a chat rather than just dealing with the professional bits.

As concerns the practice, I've probably seen about twenty community nurses in these three and a half years. I don't think, when people are referred, they seem to understand the role of the community nurse. There's an expectation … if you live round here, they expect a good service. And the demands that are put on the practice here are, in some respects, quite unreasonable. And I think it should be explained why they're not having home visits. The concept of community nursing, I would suggest, is not understood as well as it should be.

I'm going off a little bit my experience as a patient, but I can't divorce the two totally. The patient participation group [at the GP practice] that I chair, last year we initiated a rolling together of all the agencies round here. Now, what we have got round here is a tremendous lot of agencies. You know, if there's an area in the whole of Great Britain with better facilities, lead me to it, because I think it's very good. But integration …

What do the patients say about how easy is it to get an appointment?

R: It's awful. You're on the phone for ages trying to get through … and they'll give you a menu of options of numbers to press, and you don't fit into it, necessarily. You're not certain – was it 3 you wanted or 4?

And getting an appointment, the communication in our surgery is awful. There's a lot of reliance on the Internet, but everyone doesn't have Internet … particularly elderly people. The practice manager seems overwhelmed, but having said that, it does need someone to be able to stand back and ask: what is going on here? Everything is done in a rush and not thought through ... for example, I was asked to book a non-urgent appointment with the doctor. I went in the morning to see the nurse, for my routine, twice a week, dressing, and when I went to reception to book the doctor's appointment, she said, you have to ring first thing in the morning. Well, but I'm there. I'm there.

You were in the surgery, and they said you have to ring?

R: Yes, I was in the surgery. There's a lack of communication between the practice reception head, and the counter itself. Communication is very important.

Now, as far as the practice pharmacist is concerned, I've had an email exchange about it. The difficulty there is that you get Pharmacist X, who is in situ, but then he goes away for a fortnight, and there's a locum. Now, the locum isn't as well qualified as the first one. As a patient, you go to the pharmacist expecting the service you got on the first occasion from the first person, but can't get the same because of depth of knowledge, or whatever it is, from the second. That's a problem ...

You must have got to know the GPs pretty well at the practice, not just because of your own health conditions, but also as chair of the PPG [patients participation group]: what is their response to the fact – because they're in charge; it's their practice – that it's so hard to get through, it's a struggle to get an appointment, and when you're in the surgery, you're told to ring; you're not allowed to actually make an appointment while you're there?

R: Being honest, I don't know, I haven't discussed it with them. Probably in the last year I've seen four different ones, but – wrongly or rightly – I haven't felt it appropriate to intrude on their time for, in a surgery appointment. And they don't come to PPG meetings.

Story 22: Rabiya

Rabiya cares for her mum, who has early-onset dementia and doesn't speak English well. The process of getting a diagnosis was protracted and placed a huge strain on Rabiya, as a young mother herself, and on her family. There were then big barriers in securing any kind of social care support. As a Muslim Asian woman, Rabiya relates multiple experiences of discrimination, and, in marked contrast, an episode of real kindness from a physiotherapist.

Rabiya: It started probably about four years ago, and at that time I worked in the NHS in mental health services. My mum had been suffering from clinical depression for a long time so I was a young carer from a very, very young age. I noticed, maybe because of me working in mental health services, that this wasn't her usual way of being; this wasn't depression. We noticed a few times that she'd been a bit forgetful: she was used to cooking for large families, we come from a very large Asian family, and she'd nearly burnt the kitchen down twice. The first time it happened we put it down as probably an accident. The second time we were a bit concerned.

My sister lives right next door to my mum and we are six children so we float in and out, but she was quite independent and I think, in Asian families, there's no such thing as living on your own because family flow in and out all the time. One of us is always staying over, but at that time I would class her as independent.

There was another occasion where she didn't realise she was putting water into hot oil … We went to the doctor's and they said, monitor it, basically. I don't think they were taking it very seriously. She was 56. Very young for dementia. Anyway, things started getting worse. She was locking herself out of the home. Luckily we live in a village-y area so the shopkeepers knew her and we had a few relatives nearby who if they saw her wandering around would telephone us, so we knew it was getting a bit serious.

It was very difficult to get a diagnosis. It took two years. All the tests were done in English. And at first it was, well, you can't translate for your mum because you're a relative. I knew about NHS policies and procedures so I said, okay, let's bring a translator in. It took ages to organise a translator, a day where I could take time off work and Mum could be available and a translator could be available. Mum had started to withdraw at this point because of everything that was going on, and I said, she won't communicate with a stranger. I mean, it takes a lot of effort to even get her into the appointment. So we tried a couple of times with the translator. It just didn't work.

So this went back and forth for a long time and we just couldn't get a diagnosis. At one point I said, why don't you have the translator there who could listen to what I'm translating to Mum because she will respond to me, but I was still not allowed to translate. Eventually it got to a point where I unfortunately had to be quite assertive. I don't like to be aggressive or assertive but I was getting really frustrated. I was really concerned about Mum. I've got a sister working in law, one in the police. I'm the only one working in the healthcare system so they were looking to me to get support for Mum. I work in the system and I couldn't navigate it. How frustrating is that?

Eventually we found a consultant who was willing to take us a little bit seriously. He was Asian so he could understand where I was coming from. I felt like he understood me better and it wasn't like I was fighting the system to get a diagnosis for Mum. We eventually did and the diagnosis, through tests, was done. She didn't just have Alzheimer's, she also had vascular dementia, and she was given the medication of memantine, which she is still on now. My frustration with the system is Mum could have been on that two years ago. It wasn't just because of the translation, it was also because they were unwilling to accept that she could have dementia at such a young age.

Now whilst this was going on I was basically doing an assessment at home constantly. It put an enormous amount of pressure on myself, on my family. I had a young child at the time as well. It was very, very stressful. I felt not heard by the system and I feel like sometimes – and I work in the system so I understand it – the system doesn't listen to the people who are doing the care. Well, maybe that was a one-off. Oh, well, we can't diagnose her if she can't speak English. All of these things are something wrong with the system rather than something wrong with my mum. She should be able to get her care. So I think that's a massive health inequality there.

Our GP, I've known him since we moved to the area in 1998. Even to this day our relationship is, I would say, quite strained because he was not willing to listen to me and I had to bypass him and he did not take that well. My GP was very resistant to diagnose, but instead of trying to seek another way to deal with the problem, they just said, we can't do the test. I felt that it was too complicated and he didn't want to deal with it because it wasn't a straightforward process.

I did put a formal complaint against the GP and I feel it's unfair that I was put in that position. I feel it's unfair that I had to complain about him and take it to all levels to get care for Mum; it's an unnecessary additional stress. That's not even including the emotional stress and the state of us when we did get that diagnosis and we knew there was something wrong with Mum. To this day I don't think I fully emotionally processed that I'm slowly losing my mum every day because I'm just on caring mode whenever I'm with her because the system isn't very supportive of allowing me that space to do that because I don't get help from the system. I feel like I'm fighting the system regularly. All the time.

Is your mum still living in her own home?

R: Yes, my brothers had to move in. The consultant who made the diagnosis was excellent. He said, we don't know how soon it will be that she'll lose capacity to consent, so I advise you to get legal-appointed status. Through his guidance I got legal power of attorney for health and finances, so out of our family, I'm the one that does all the care arrangements. Me and my younger sister, who lives next door, do her personal care and my brothers do the shopping, feeding and other stuff. Because of our cultural upbringing, my mum would not allow my brothers to support her with her personal care.

I felt more comfortable talking to the hospital consultant who was Asian, saying to him, yes, we are in the home all the time with Mum, you know what it's like with Asian families, this is how we are. We've noticed the change, and it wasn't that I had to prove myself. He just accepted it whilst with the GP, who is white, I felt like constantly I had to prove, when did it happen? Suddenly because I can't put a date, time and log of when it happened he's like, well, did it really happen? He started questioning me. I was the one that was interrogated. It was unnecessary. It put more stress on me.

The hospital consultant was very helpful. He said, one thing you might want to consider is what impact this might have on her physical state and whether you guys can support. We all work full-time so we all had to manage the care around our jobs. He said, you might want to seek support from social services. Even though I work in the healthcare system I didn't know enough about the social care at that time, so I rang all the relevant numbers. It took ages for someone to come out and do an assessment, months.

Eventually I had to go back to the GP and ask them to refer to the social services because we couldn't do a direct referral, for whatever reason. I think I might have even gone back to the consultant and asked him to write a letter and he was very supportive. When the social worker came over, she was a lovely lady, I still can remember her face. She went through the social care assessment and she asked who was supporting the care and I said, well, right now we all are but we wanted to see what was available. I'm really worried, especially about the touch point during the day when we're all at work, whether she'd be all right at home alone and I'm a bit concerned about that. So they said, well, we can provide carers to come in and do some touch points. I was like, oh, right, okay, so Mum doesn't speak English so it would have to be someone that can communicate in Bengali because, especially with her dementia, she gets withdrawn really, really quickly, and they said, we can't guarantee that.

I was like, oh, okay, right, well, I don't think that's going to work then because she will feel very afraid and she might react towards that. I said, okay, can you make sure it's going to be a woman? She said, no, we can't guarantee that either. I said, well, my mum is a survivor of domestic violence. My dad was very, very physically violent towards her so if you're telling me that a random person – they said, they can't even be consistent with who arrives – so you're saying a random person, who could be a bloke, could arrive at her home, let himself in, that's just not going to work. It's going to put her in such a state. She doesn't even let her sons as men come near her.

There followed a conversation about Rabiya's mum's earlier life.

R: My dad moved abroad to Bangladesh. At the point he left was when I was in secondary school and that's when Mum got diagnosed with clinical depression. It all deteriorated then. My younger brother and sister were still at home, so I was caring for them and caring for Mum at the same time.

Basically Mum got diagnosed with clinical depression and that was it. She was just on tablets. To be honest, thinking back now, I am surprised that no further questions were asked, especially when there were three children at home under the age of 16 – I was 14. Mum was on her own by then, and my older three siblings had already left home by then.

So your mum's had a really hard life, hasn't she?

R: Yes, and with that comes all the kind of cultural kind of expectations of women as well. So the way my mum's been brought up, it's been the woman who feeds and looks after the family, et cetera. There is a deference to men. I mean, that is the reality whether I accept it or not, whether I agree with it or not, that is the reality, so there are certain things my mum would not ask her sons to do, even though they would be willing to. When I realised we couldn't get any carer support, and the social worker was very direct about it, and I'd prefer her to be direct about it, but once again, I was quite frustrated with the system because I thought, to be honest, if we're talking truly about individualising person-centred care, you basically are saying: a) my mum couldn't get a diagnosis for a number of years and b) now you're saying she can't get care because the system is not set up to support her in that sense. And there was no personal budget option.

Rabiya goes on to talk about caring for her mum after the diagnosis of dementia.

R: At that time also caring for Mum was getting quite intensive. I was going through quite a difficult period because my siblings were at the point where they were not willing to accept the diagnosis, so I was doing the majority of the care. It was having an impact on going to work. It was having an impact on spending quality time with my daughter. It was having an impact on my health as well.

At that time, the new carer's assessment started coming through. So someone came out from the local authority and I said, well, it's quite horrific, to be honest, I feel like, as a carer, I know it's my responsibility to look after Mum, but I feel like how can the system expect me to work, pay taxes, look after my own home, look after Mum's home and pay the bills – that's just a practical aspect. I have a young child, I'm a single parent and manage all that and then look after Mum to a level where she can have a good quality of life herself. It's very contradictory and it's not supportive at all. Bless her, again the lady was very, very nice, and she was like, yes, that sounds really hard, okay, thank you very much, and off they went. They did direct me to the carers' centre but all the activities happen during the day when I'm at work. And, to be honest, I think sometimes when you're at that state you just want to be able to vent, just venting is quite therapeutic.

Around about that point, two years ago, we had a family meeting, and I just said, you guys are just going to have to pull your socks up, and that's when my brothers said, right, we will move in with Mum so we can be there all the time.

And my brothers started picking up the medication. They've been taking her to the standard appointments. It's become quite tick-boxy. I got a letter through the other day saying, your mum's due her annual dementia check. So I took time off work to take Mum in to do this five-minute dementia check which does nothing. It's just a tick-box. What I really needed, the last time I went to the GP, was a referral to the physiotherapy team because Mum needed a new walking stick and a referral to the incontinence team.

I can't go direct to either of these services. I have to go through a referral from the GP. So I need to take time off work, go to the GP …

It's a pain because the care gets delayed further because the GP doesn't have the appointment when I'm available. I'm not available all the time because I work. If my siblings go in, the GP doesn't give them what they need. I have to go in and then I have to be quite directive and say, okay, Dr So-and-So, useless appointment, wasted your time, I just need a referral. That's exactly what I want. I don't want to talk about anything, just do a referral. Then he makes a referral. It gets clogged in the system. The incontinence referral letter got lost. It took another three weeks …

It got to a point where I was in tears, one day when I was talking to the incontinence team administrator, and I said, I can't do this anymore, forget it. I will just buy Mum whatever she needs. I just need you to tell me based on her previous assessment what. I think the lady felt really sorry for me and she said, don't worry, we've done a previous assessment on her about two years ago … So they provided me with the pads but again, I felt like I had to not navigate the system, I had to go underhand again. Similar to the diagnosis, I had to literally beg or cry or get something done.

Have you got an example where the system has actually worked?

R: Trying to get an appointment to physiotherapy was hell, but last week, on Thursday, I took Mum to the physiotherapy appointment in a new care centre and again, whenever it's a new place, Mum is really jittery. Two appointments had been booked before but she was not in a good state. I couldn't get her out. The other thing about appointments with services – let me just quickly say this so I don't forget – if you cancel an appointment they get really arsey with you but I say to them, when my mum has dementia if I know she's in a poor mental health state, there's no point in me bringing her to the appointment because she will not engage. She won't even get in the car for me.

Sometimes I say, do you do home visits, because you coming into that space I can manage it because it's a familiar surrounding, I can calm her down, I can talk her … because she's deteriorated over the past four years so sometimes depending on her state in the morning, she'll act quite childlike and sometimes she'll be completely fine. They don't. So I said, fine, so I eventually made it to the physiotherapist and her name is Lily. I won't forget her name because she was such an amazing person.

When she asked me the questions and I said, I can't answer that because she's got dementia so I need you to consider her physical as well as her mental state, Lily got it just like that. She said, I have worked with dementia patients before, I understand. So when Lily said, how mobile is she, has her mobility deteriorated, and I said, it depends on her mental state. Some days she just won't move at all so her mobility will be zero. Other days, if it's a bright sunny day and she's in a good mood I can get her to walk a little bit longer and can get her to move around. She's got osteoporosis and arthritis as well, quite bad and during winter periods it gets worse.

She's in a lot of pain and Lily just got it. I didn't have to justify what I was saying. She just understood. She just listened to me and she said,

I understand. I remember she got a walking stick out and it was one of those hospital walking sticks, the grey ones, and my mum looked at it and she said, I'm not having that old woman stick. She was obviously saying it in Bengali to me. I was like, oh, gosh, how can I say to Lily that she doesn't want that stick? I'm really sorry, Lily, I know this is going to sound really childish but her previous stick was black, can she get a black stick? Lily was like, oh, yes, I just was recommending this one because she can use it on either hand. I completely understand, yes, no worries. If she thinks it's an old woman's stick, that's completely understandable … and she was just so supportive.

She just understood without challenging me about everything, which I feel like a lot of healthcare professionals do, to be honest. She just went and got the black stick. Mum then was quite happy with that and she responded well, so when Lily was doing some of the exercises with her she was laughing along with Mum, engaging with her. Mum didn't understand what she was saying but Mum could tell from her body language she was being supportive and she just responded really well and it put me at ease as well. I said, do we need to come for another appointment? She said, not unless you need to. If you need to, just contact the physiotherapy team direct. You don't need to come through the GP. I was like, that's great, that's so fantastic, and she said, if you need any advice or something, just give me a bell and we can have a chat over the phone if you don't want to bring your mum in. I just thought that was just really good.

I've not had to contact Lily again, but I feel like, if I do, I've got her name, number … it's very rare through my mum's healthcare journey that I can pinpoint individuals that have been really supportive. The consultant is number one and Lily is probably number two.

To what extent do you think it is about your mum's ethnic background, the fact she doesn't speak English and your ethnic background, or to what extent do you think it's the kind of hopelessness of the system that is just not joined up?

R: I think attitudes and behaviours are very, very important. My husband is white. My husband is a lovely white, middle-class, very posh-speaking Oxford-educated A&E doctor. The way people respond to him and the way they respond to me is different. I was prepared to go into that physiotherapy appointment already on guard and it was beautiful just to feel that I didn't have to be on guard and all it took was Lily to introduce herself and she goes, how are you doing? I was like, oh, how am I doing? Do you mean, Mum? She goes, no, how are you doing? I was like, oh, right, I'm a bit exhausted, I had to take this day off again. This is the third time I've tried to get her out. She just listened to me and then when she started to ask me the questions she was truly listening.

I felt like the system isn't set up to be inclusive in the services it provides to its diverse communities. I think there's almost a tightrope, being, do people think I play the race card all the time or is the system institutionally racist? People like my mum do not have access to the healthcare that people who are white will have access to because of the blockers in the system. So if we're not actively doing something to remove those barriers, we are enforcing the racist behaviour of the system.

Sometimes I go to appointments with Mum in my work clothes with my NHS lanyard on because I think I will be taken more seriously. Isn't that sad? Isn't it sad that I need to perform my professional role in order to get the care for my mum? But I do, and I feel I do because I know I'll get a better response.

One of the things that we've spoken about as a family is, what are we going to do as Mum gets older? Now in our culture, this is going to sound harsh, we don't put people in homes. We look after our elderly. Western society isn't set up to support family members. In Bangladesh the entire village will look after. It's a community thing.

Now, thankfully, Mum's got six kids. I think about all those people that don't have families and what will happen with them. There's at least four of us that can support Mum on a day-to-day basis and that's what we've just accepted that that's the way it's going to be. We've accepted that we probably won't get any support from the state that can support Mum, and we've accepted that as she gets older, we will need to rearrange our lives to make sure that we can look after her. Of course that puts strain on the relationships because, for example, I could not move away. So if I decided to get a job in Scotland I can't. We have to coordinate how we take holidays.

I think there is an assumption made that because Mum comes from an Asian background, she'll have family to look after her.

The conversation then turned to support from the GP practice.

R: If you were to ask me, is there anyone that I feel like I've connected with in the healthcare system that really sees Mum as an individual or has taken responsibility about supporting me in her care, I would say no.

She's borderline diabetic, so about every six months I need to go and have her bloods checked. She also has low blood pressure so sometimes if her blood levels are not right she passes out and she also has a rotary tear. So every six months she needs to go and have some steroid injections. It's very difficult when it feels like you are having to navigate five or six different services at any one given time and every one of them feels like there's a problem with it. Now, it's not always the healthcare professional themselves, but getting to the healthcare professional can be a problem.

Story 23: James

We first met James in Chapter 2 when he related his experiences of becoming a dad, and how he and his partner fared during childbirth and afterwards. Before that, James looked after his mother for ten years after her diagnosis of dementia until she died. He set up a carers' support group in his local area because he found there wasn't much help and support. This enabled James and his mum to enjoy outings and holidays. After his mum had a spell in hospital which made her largely bedbound, the local health and social care agencies very efficiently arranged home care support. The care provider didn't always provide the level of care that had been commissioned and James had to push to get that put right. There were a couple of episodes towards the end of his mum's life which stand out for James which are a reminder about the need to plan ahead.

James: My dad had died when I was 17. He'd had cancer, so that was quite tough. My sister was 15. Mum was still young. She really loved my dad and she didn't want to meet anyone else because the time she had with him was really special. She didn't have that need to meet anyone else.

And then we started noticing things. The same month that my mum was diagnosed with Alzheimer's and dementia, my employer asked me to relocate down south. I thought, I can't really do that, she's in her hour of need, so I'll take redundancy. That was probably ten or eleven years ago now. I was 42 then. She didn't want to go in a care home, so I said, I'll do as much as I can to prevent that.

My sister said that she couldn't be a carer, it's not her nature. You save for a rainy day and it started drizzling a bit so I thought, right, it's payback time. She looked after me fantastically well as a little lad, great mother, I couldn't hope for a better mum, I need to look after her.

When she became incontinent, and as she deteriorated, she needed me there all the time. So, I rented out my house and moved in with Mum. My sister was at work. I got weekends off occasionally, so she would look after her …

It worked quite well. My sister did things like bathing her and I did everything else. I maintained her dignity. She became incontinent, but I could still manage to maintain her dignity, believe it or not. It was only until the last six months of her life, when she was in bed all the time. I felt I couldn't do that. There were things I couldn't do as a son for my mum, really. That's my mum.

She was 64 when she was diagnosed. I was absolutely astonished at how poorly she'd performed in a simple memory test. It was a real eye-opener for me when she couldn't draw the numbers around a face of a clock. It was a wake-up call, really because you just think some of these things are because she's getting a bit older.

When she was diagnosed, I was disappointed with the service she got from the NHS. It was a case of, right, there's your diagnosis, you've got mixed dementia, Alzheimer's and vascular dementia, here's some tablets, come back in twelve months, and that's it. This is a massive, life-changing thing for her and for her family. We didn't know what to expect. So I whizzed up to the library to get all the books I can on dementia and Alzheimer's. All the books I could get were clinical. Where's the help about how we help her to live?

We just cracked on with it. Mum was doing okay. Then she started falling out of bed a lot. You'd just hear a massive crash during the night, she'd be on the floor. Then she became quite challenging and we had to look out for help from somewhere. Then we became aware of the carers' centre. The support there was excellent. There was a carer's assessment as well, which was great. On the back of that, we were referred to occupational therapists and they got the council to come out and fix a fantastic bit of kit. Just on the wall, and it had like an infrared beam round her bed, so that if ever she put her leg over it, an alarm would go off and it would prevent her from hurting herself by falling out of bed. You could just run and help her.

Alzheimer's Society was there as a support group. The thing about that was you were not allowed to take the person you cared for – it was only for carers – so what do you do with the person that you care for? Also, we weren't allowed to bring the cared-for person with you to the Christmas dinner, which everyone was devastated by. So, I thought, this isn't right. Everything's about risk and you couldn't do anything with the person with dementia.

We thought, right, we need something better than this. So, we set up a charitable group and we'll work round these risks. We took everyone out for a Christmas meal. That was eight years ago now and it really took off. We had good support from the older people's psychologist at the local specialist mental health service. She had a real passion to create a group like this for years. There's no staff, there's no employees, it's all goodwill. We take people on holiday once a year. It's fab. Mum loved that. It doesn't matter if you embarrass yourself because everyone's in the same ...

The conversation then turned to support from the GP practice.

J: I was worried about power of attorney and her capacity and also her health. The GP just said, I haven't got time for that, your appointment is only ten minutes. That was all. So, he wasn't very helpful at all.

At the time, it was a case of, well you've got your diagnosis, just get on with it, really. There was no support whatever. It was only towards the end of her life, when she was on the end-of-life pathway, where the GP got more actively involved. In fact, the GPs were very good. They'd come out frequently because she got infections and things like that.

But in that ten-year time, she was hardly ever at the GP, which I suppose, physically, she was okay. But she had trouble with incontinence. That was a real difficult time. She was doubly incontinent, ultimately, but initially it was just urine that she was incontinent. A gap there was no one tells you how long you should keep a pad on or what it looks like when it's full. Then you think, well, we're not getting enough pads here to cope with her needs. Then it's a case of, well, we only supply that many. So, it's like, right, what are we doing wrong here? So, in the end, the NHS would supply so many pads a week and we just went out and bought whatever we needed.

I did think the education side to the carer could be a lot better on managing incontinence for her. Another thing that was a problem was your bin gets full very quickly. You have to apply to the council for another bin and people don't tell you about these things.

What happened with the support, it came in dribs and drabs. You had the falls team who came in when she fell. That was a real harrowing time, when she'd fall and hurt herself, because her spatial awareness deteriorated as she went along. For example, if you had a change in the carpet somewhere, she would freeze and you'd have to show her that you can actually make that step onto that different carpet. Or even on the pavement. I remember taking her somewhere for a meal and there was a shadow on the floor in the pavement, at night-time, and she thought it was a hole ... she was petrified of taking that step.

She fell and she had a fracture on her wrist. That was awful for her 'cause she lost her ability to use a knife and fork then. These little aids that came in, like a commode, it wasn't really joined up, there wasn't like a plan. It was just like, if something happened, you had to think, who do I ask about this, who do I go to?

I could live off my savings, basically, so it didn't really matter. But I did feel a bit aggrieved that this is a chunk of my life that I'm giving Mum. She deserves it. But you do think, oh, gosh, what will I do after this? On a bit of a scrapheap, sort of thing. So, it's a worry. And I had cabin fever big time. You go from quite a demanding job to that and it's like, oh my goodness.

I thought, I'll volunteer for the NHS so that when people have just received a diagnosis of dementia, me as a carer and the psychiatric nurse will have an informal chat with them to tell them what's available, for about an hour, to an hour and a half. I produced a checklist of everything to discuss with them, like power of attorney, support groups, the carers' centre, benefits, and all the rest of it. We did that for some years.

Something that was really sad for Mum, she soon formed pressure ulcers on her hips when she was at home and I do think that could have been avoided. They got to category-4 pressure ulcers and they were really bad. Eventually, they got a special mattress for her. I thought, there's no way will they ever heal up. I mean, fair play to the district nurses, they perfectly healed. They were absolutely amazing what they did with her. But if that could have been avoided, it would have saved the NHS so much time, effort. So, the preventative side, maybe they could have given her a mattress straightaway, or told me, look, you need to think about getting this mattress because she's at risk of this.

I felt like I'd let her down there because this had happened and they could have prevented that. You think of the time and effort for those district nurses to come and do that for months and months.

In the August, she had cellulitis in her leg, which meant she had to go into hospital and they put her on antibiotics. She's in there for probably about six or eight weeks. I was there every day with her. She couldn't really talk much, and the food would come, the plate in front of her, and then she was left to do it. So, I had to go in and feed her, every mealtime.

I stayed with her all day and then my sister would go after she'd been to work, for an hour. That's when they said, look, she can't mobilise now, she's going to go home and stay in her bed, basically. So, she had a hospital bed at home with a mattress that moved to prevent her getting pressure ulcers. Then she got a package of care.

What was excellent was when she was discharged from hospital, everything worked fantastically well in terms of the staff at the hospital. The council's social workers arranged that package of care so quickly and so well and got the bed in there, got a care company who would come out ... 'cause she had to be moved for her pressure ulcers as well – four times a day, I think it was. They'd come in four times a day, move her, change her dressings, et cetera. She lasted another six months.

Then one day, she was very ill. I got up in the morning, she was obviously in distress and she'd been sick, like coffee grounds or something like that, 999. Then it's a case of, right, she's on a DNR [do not resuscitate order] anyway, which she agreed she wanted? But they did anyway take her to A&E, they were fab. They couldn't even take any blood 'cause her blood pressure was so low and ... beepers going off all over the place. She came through again, and she got home and then lasted another three months at home.

So, what difference did it make to you and your sister when you found that the care was so well organised between the hospital and social care?

J: The healthcare professional and the social worker met with me and my sister in the hospital together. While Mum was in there, the social worker had done a lot of fact-finding about our situation. Then on the actual day of discharge we met there and talked about what's going to happen. Everything that they said would happen, happened. I was amazed. It was just like, wow, this is so good. We'd had nothing before. We can actually go out, and things like that, and not worry about Mum, she's going to be all right.

Although it was fantastic at the start, what we soon found ... She was commissioned to have two carers, first thing in the morning, lunchtime, about five o'clock, and then ten o'clock at night. Frequently, you'd find either only one carer would turn up ... there should be two people to move her safely ... or there might be no one turn up. That's when I thought, someone's paying for this and we're not getting the service that we've been expecting here. So, a few times I marched off to the care provider and said, well, this is not on.

The ladies who were providing the care was fantastic, they were rushed off their feet, they always did a great job, we got to know them well. It was just poor management or not enough staff, basically, at the care provider. But when you keep banging on about it to them, she got what she was entitled to, but only because I kept going on. If you were a carer who hasn't got that time or capacity to do that, you could be walked all over.

Can I ask about – if it's not too hard and difficult – what it was like in the last few days of her life?

J: The district nurses started coming in a bit more frequently. For Mum, it was the same, playing music for her, talking to her. At the end I used to give her fluids by a syringe, to keep her lips moistened all the time 'cause they were very dry. Food, she would just have anything that was full of sugar, basically. Her swallow wasn't very good. So everything had to be thickened. Then it was just keeping her hydrated and with some amount of food. But the last three days or so, that wasn't important. The nurses said, don't worry about that. What is important is about keeping her comfortable. There were all these drugs prescribed that were sat in a cupboard waiting and they had to be checked every now and again. At the end she was put on a syringe drive with morphine. Literally, that was in the morning and then she passed away by two o'clock.

One thing I would have done differently is for me and my sister to sit down and discuss what we both wanted for her death. Because I made the assumption that my sister would want to be there with Mum when it finally happened, wrongly, and she didn't want to do that. I was on the phone to her, saying, look, this is it, you've got to get here as quick as you can. Of course, she starts crying. I was thinking, gosh, you've got to get here, I don't want you to miss her and the chance to say goodbye. Whereas I didn't know that she was happy with how we'd left it. If we'd have had that discussion, I wouldn't have been in as much of a flap at the time.

Story 24: Sheila

Sheila cares for her husband, who has dementia. She describes the battle to get a diagnosis and care in place with little support from the GP. They used her husband's private medical insurance to access medical consultant advice and monitoring.

Sheila: He is 85 ... he has been diagnosed with dementia, probably Alzheimer's, and now secondarily with Parkinson's disease ... he's been diagnosed more than ten years. When we first went to the GP he clearly felt I was worrying unnecessarily and that the concerns I was expressing were normal for a then 74-, 75-year-old as in forgetfulness, and reluctance to get engaged with the activities that he used to perform quite comfortably. So I got nowhere with that, so I had to invent another symptom.

I gave new life to previous symptoms that Brian had had. He had problems with his heart, he had atrial fibrillation and he hadn't had any episodes for a few years, but I felt that this was another route into further exploration. So I took him back to the doctor and said I was concerned that he was having increasing heart problems and wondered if there was something could be done. It was at that point that he was sent off for testing and he was diagnosed.

Later on there was a crisis in which he fell over and dislocated his shoulder. At that point we ended up within the radar of social services and at that point I was aware that there were resources I could tap into. Everything that I've discovered, I've discovered on my own. I didn't know who the gatekeepers were, the signposters. I now am aware that there are useful people but I often discovered them fairly randomly: an article in the local paper offering some sort of carers' support … coffee meeting, for instance … which I attended and then found there were other resources that I could access via a very efficient carers' forum. It's all been really random.

I became aware of things like memory clinics, which I understand is a sort of euphemism for a general one-stop shop, which I heard about and I thought would be quite useful to go and check that out. I did think it was good as a one-stop shop because you saw a nurse, a physio, an OT [occupational therapist], who all gave you the big picture. I thought it was jolly useful. But logistically it was a nightmare. The local hospital were having repairs done at the time. I had to drop B off in his wheelchair at the entrance and then drive for ages to park. By the time I got back, somebody had moved Brian. So we didn't do it again. The logistics were too much. But it was, you know, I thought there was potential. But we did have a private consultant who met some of the broader needs or certainly was more able to signpost.

Is it the same GP that you've had all this time?

S: We changed the practice only a couple of years ago when we moved to a new location. Brian had had that previous GP for some years. I think I could say we had no support from the GP. Brian was very fit and healthy; we rarely needed to see them again. Having got ourselves into the system and found a very good private consultant, we were then a bit out of the loop. I can't remember really going back to the GP after that, although I did get an amazing letter at one point from the practice asking me to rate the support that I was being offered by the practice in relation to being a carer for my husband … I had to reply to that: no support, what support?

However, the new practice then made a new appointment. Something like patient coordinator, who came visiting us at home, spent an hour with us filling in the form, and I felt she had a great potential to be very useful and certainly it felt that this would be a very useful channel for me. I have actually used her a couple of times. I phoned her up when I needed advice, information, help, and although didn't have the answer then, was very prompt in getting back to me ... I felt there finally was someone who I could just ring up and ask for support. Yes.

Story 25: Kauri

Kauri's dad died recently of pancreatic cancer. There had been some delay in getting a diagnosis, which was finally made after a second visit to A&E. Kauri goes on to narrate many episodes of excellent care and support given by the hospital and the GP, including a three-month hospital stay and end-of-life care supported by district nurses, visiting hospice staff and GP. The main challenge for Kauri as the prime carer was managing the differing demands of the wider family during this difficult time.

Kauri: In March last year, my dad was diagnosed with pancreatic cancer. He had been suffering with symptoms from October, mostly to do with sickness, nausea, and that had got progressively worse. He did go to see the GP in October, because he was complaining of pain in his back. They did an ultrasound, there was nothing obvious showing. He just thought that he was on his feet quite a lot. He was a picture framer, so he was very active in terms of this job, and he just thought that he was wearing the wrong footwear, and it was getting cold so he just put his back pain down to a few other related issues. The sickness got worse, so we got to a point where after eating he would have to go and be sick because he just couldn't keep the food down. The period of time between sickness got shorter and shorter. He went for a number of tests as an outpatient in December and January and they didn't show anything untoward. On 15 February he was very ill and was being sick a lot during the day and my younger brother decided that it was just ridiculous: he needed to go to A&E. He'd actually been to A&E two weeks before and they hadn't found anything and had suggested that he just carried on with the tests that had been arranged through an outpatient appointment.

So Dad went into hospital on 15 February, and he stayed in hospital for three months. It took a month to diagnose, and that was because of the position of the tumour. The endoscopy and the colonoscopy showed nothing. The initial CT scan didn't show a great deal, so a biopsy was done, but because the area was so inflamed the results of the first biopsy weren't very clear at all. So we had to wait and completely clear the stomach so that a second biopsy could be done. All through this time Dad wasn't eating. So from 15 February he wasn't eating at all. He was drinking a little bit but no food was being consumed. It was a very scary time for him. He was not used to being in hospital at all. He had run his own business for thirty-seven years and was very used to being in his shop, in his little community, very well respected, very well liked. So to go from that to being in a hospital bed was just a complete shock to the system. It was a complete shock to all of us as well.

He was 68 at the time. It turned our lives upside down as well. I was very fortunate that I could work from home and be very flexible in terms of what I did and take time off. My younger brother took time off from his job as well and started picking up bits and pieces at the shop, because we'd still got a pipeline of customer work.

And most of our customers are very understanding. They still have pieces of work that they want to give us, gifts or something, so we needed to keep on top of that, so myself and my younger brother did that. Mum was just very concerned about what was going on. The care overall that he was receiving was good, but it was very frustrating because we didn't know what was happening. I took it on myself to be the point person for the family and the consultants. I would go to the hospital on a daily basis outside of visiting hours so that I could see the consultant and be there when the consultant did their rounds with Dad.

Dad was very clear that he wanted somebody to be with him, and the consultants got to know us quite well because literally the minute visiting time started I was there and I was there throughout, and when Dad was first admitted he was on a gastro ward, and I think visiting was something like twelve till seven, so it was for the majority of the day. I just asked, can we come in and talk to the consultants? And they said yes. They were very accommodating in that respect, and Dad was in a bay of four, so he wasn't in a side room or anything. But we were still very aware that there were other patients around, so after the consultant had done their rounds we'd have a little chat and then we'd go off and get a coffee or something and Dad would have a little snooze, because he wasn't sleeping very well. We weren't there as a permanent fixture, but we did make a point of being at the hospital at about nine, 9:30 every day in the morning, so that we could catch consultants.

It made a huge difference for Dad. It really reassured him. My dad speaks English, he understands English very well. But it just helped him knowing that there was somebody else there listening. And I would always make a point of making sure that Dad had understood what the consultants were saying. The consultants would talk to Dad, and if they talked to me I would direct them to talk to Dad, because I'm just there as a secondary, I'm just there to listen. I would always make sure that Dad understood and had the opportunity to ask any questions, so it didn't become a conversation with me as his daughter; it was still a conversation with Dad as the patient, I was just there to help and support him. We'd have a little think beforehand if there were results of a test that we didn't understand or something, and we'd have a little chat beforehand and we'd write down some questions. So I constantly carried a notebook around with me, and encouraged Dad to write down questions when they came to his mind as well so he didn't forget them.

I probably know most of the consultant gastroenterologists at the hospital now, and they were all very accommodating, very helpful. One in particular who did the biopsies, who came to tell Dad the results of the second biopsy, was very interested in Dad's care, to the point that he wasn't the consultant on ward that week but he still came with the consultant who was looking after the ward to give Dad the results of the biopsy, because he also wanted to get to the bottom of it. At first they thought it was a treatable cancer, but once they did the second biopsy they understood that it was pancreatic. They didn't tell us the stage at the time, but then I spoke to the clinical director who was on ward rounds the week that we found out Dad's diagnosis, and he was very direct with me and basically said stage three, nearly stage four, you're looking at three to six months. So in terms of sharing a message with me they were very direct, probably because they knew I could handle it. They were still direct with Dad. When we had the diagnosis – I will never forget that. Mum, my aunt, me and Dad, in the cubicle with the curtain drawn, so, interestingly, not in a separate room. Other patients could hear. And we were devastated, obviously. At that point I think I just had to put the diagnosis to one side because I'd got family really annoying me to be honest.

Wider family asking constant questions. I've got an aunt and uncle in the States who are clinicians and they were constantly asking to speak to the consultants here and I was saying no, because they're not oncologists. My uncle's a GP who specialises in diabetes, and my aunt's a diabetes nurse, so – sorry, no. There's probably a lot of relationships in my wider family that won't be the same, won't be as open, won't be as engaging, because I was very clear from the start that any conversations about Dad's care included Dad. So there were no side conversations with the consultants and anybody else who might have a medical interest or background or experience. Because, as far as I'm concerned, Dad's the patient, this is happening to Dad, it's not happening to anybody else, so if that conversation doesn't include Dad, then it's not happening.

And how was your mum, as the other very close person to your dad, with that approach that you took?

K: My youngest brother and my mum were completely supportive. My other brother less so. He had his own agendas. He took it upon himself to communicate to the wider family when we didn't even know what was going on, so we weren't ready to share information, whereas he was the first one to pick up the phone. And that continued.

Our family is practising Sikh. There's a very large Sikh community in XXX. Really helpfully, some of the nurses speak a little bit of Punjabi to be able to converse with their patients. That was really nice for Dad to hear. There was one male nurse in particular on one of the surgical wards that Dad was on and he would converse in Punjabi, and Dad would teach him correct pronunciations. There were other Sikh patients on the ward that would get to know Dad, and actually Dad was able to converse with them when their English might have not been so good. So he was there to help translate ...

The hospital knew that I was always the one there to help them with any questions about Dad. They also knew that if I asked any questions they were genuine questions, and I was collating information and trying to get answers. He had two stomach bypasses. Dad's main concern was that he couldn't eat, and so – regardless of anything else – he wanted to be able to eat. So the consultant agreed to do a stomach bypass. That basically replumbed through into the stomach so that they bypassed where the tumour was.

Unfortunately the first bypass didn't work as well. So only five weeks after the first operation Dad had a second more complicated bypass. And then two days after that he haemorrhaged. I'm convinced that it was partly due to the stress of having wider family come and visit. Dad always put other people first. So family would come and visit and his main concern would be, so what are you going to eat tonight? Make sure you eat, don't leave without us feeding you. They'd come to visit him and he would be more concerned about making sure that as a family we were hospitable and looking after them.

I have an aunt and uncle who live in Kent, they're very unsteady on their feet. They insisted on coming and visiting but would not let me know in advance. So on the day that he haemorrhaged they turned up, and we'd told people that he was undergoing surgery. He's two days after having a second major stomach operation, he's not up to visitors. He got so, so upset. He sat down with my aunt, she was in tears, he was in tears, and he said, look, this is not right, you can pick up the phone and talk to me, you do not have to come and see me, this is not helping. And that evening he haemorrhaged.

We rushed back to the hospital. The ward wouldn't let us in. They knew that we were there. One of the nurses, she was just doing her job, but she could have probably been a little bit more empathetic. And we could hear him. We could hear him being ill, and I was trying to ring the ward to find out what was going on as we were driving, and the ward telephone had been given, coincidentally, to the man in the next bed as my dad. A patient answered the ward phone. This is probably at about 9:30 at night. Bless him, he said, oh, I'm really sorry, the ward staff are dealing with an emergency so they're a little bit stretched. I said, yes, I think that emergency is my dad.

We probably waited outside the ward window for about an hour. They let Mum in first, then they let me and my younger brother in, and every five minutes or so Dad was throwing up blood. It was awful. The trust instigated their major haemorrhage procedure. One of the nurses on the ward was very young and afterwards she said that this was the first time she'd ever been involved in anything so serious. It seemed like it took forever for the on-call gastroenterologist to appear, and it was somebody we'd never seen, and she was umm-ing and ah-ing and Dad was like, you need to do something, I'm in a lot of pain here. Some useless junior doctor appeared to take blood from Dad to work out what his blood group was, and in the meantime Dad's saying, I'm AB positive, I'm AB positive. Because they decided at that point he needed a transfusion.

And all of this – it's probably like eleven o'clock at night – the rest of the patients in the ward are trying to sleep but there's all this commotion going on. And they can hear everything. So Dad's not moved to a side room or somewhere a bit quieter, this is all on a bay with probably five or six patients. Dad ended up going in for an emergency procedure. He had eight units of blood that evening. He went to ICU. It was probably the longest evening of our lives. We literally stayed at the hospital all night-long whilst he was in surgery, and then waiting for him to be taken into ICU. Luckily he was transferred out of ICU back onto the surgical ward into a side rom the following day. Only two weeks after that he was discharged home, after a three-month stay. He went in on 15 February, he came out on 15 May.

In general, the consultants were very accommodating with our requests, which personally was very helpful. So I didn't have any battles. The nurses, in the week, during the day, absolutely fantastic in terms of the number of nurses available and the response time if Dad needed something. At night and at the weekends Dad would say that he could tell that they were doing their absolute best, but they were stretched.

There were some nurses that Dad liked more than others. Dad celebrated his birthday on the gastro ward on 16 March, and all the nurses organised a cake for Dad and they signed a card and they sung happy birthday to him. We were so touched. It was such a wonderfully generous thing to do. We've got a picture of all the nurses with Dad.

And he really put the effort into building that relationship with the people that looked after him.

Kauri then talked about when her dad came home after the three-month stay in hospital.

K: He was referred to a hospice for palliative care. They are absolutely fantastic. We were assigned a palliative care nurse that came to start with on a weekly basis, and she was as concerned about us as a family as she was with Dad and his care, and she made it very clear that she was there to look after all of us and support all of us. Mum and Dad's GP was very engaged as well. Mum and Dad have been at that GP practice for thirty-four years, got a really good relationship. The lead GP for palliative care was very frustrated that it had taken so long to diagnose the problem, and she made the extra effort to come and see Dad on a regular basis at home and to make sure that he was okay.

We got the impression from all of the team at the hospice, as well as the GP, that they genuinely cared about Dad and us. So between Mum and I, we looked after Dad at home. So Dad was mobile. He decided that he was going to stay in our spare room because that was nearer the bathroom for him and it meant that he would get a good night's sleep and Mum would get a good night's sleep in her room as well. So we moved a few things around and got Dad comfortable in there, and he was very self-sufficient to start with.

I took it upon myself with my youngest brother and my mum to devise a little chart of food, and we would between us manage what Dad ate, and we would try lots of different things. Some things he liked, some things he didn't. So we did whatever we could to try and encourage him to eat. And it wasn't helped by family asking questions like, do you feel hungry, so what's it like not having eaten, and clearly ridiculous questions. Some of my family have zero tact. All the time we're managing Dad coming home, we're still having to deal with the wider family who are saying he should be having chemo, and have you looked at this treatment and have you looked at that treatment. And at that time he wasn't strong enough for chemo.

We had an oncologist appointment for the end of May because they wanted to wait until Dad had fully recovered from surgery before considering options. And at that point Dad was offered a very low dose of chemo and then had an infection which meant a return to hospital.

During all of this my younger brother had proposed to his girlfriend, and they decided to bring the wedding forward to July. So whilst we were planning an Indian wedding in three weeks, we also had to deal with the fact that Dad was back in hospital again for the third time. He wasn't eating as well by now, so my ideal of six very small meals throughout the day was becoming more like three or four because Dad was sleeping a lot. We felt very guilty waking him up to give him food.

But he fully enjoyed my brother's wedding. It was in a Sikh temple. We'd arranged for a little side room, we'd taken a foldout bed, a duvet, a heater. It was in the middle of July but the weather wasn't fantastic. Dad didn't need any of that. He drew on all of the love in the room to get him through the day, and he was as proud as punch to see his youngest son get married ...

He started to have bouts of very low blood pressure, and that caused him to black out, and that was very scary for us. And all of the time we are still looking after him at home, Mum and I and my youngest brother. We are getting more support from hospice. So the palliative nurse is probably coming twice a week now. The GPs may be coming on a more regular basis to help alleviate symptoms and trying different things like increasing pain relief. So Dad's not on morphine or anything at this point. He's still on a combination of paracetamol and co-codamol, but we're just changing the combination slightly. But the dips in low blood pressure are starting to concern us. And he is sleeping a lot more. We persuaded him to have a hospital bed because it's more comfortable for him. He's very reluctant, but we persuaded him that that's the right thing to do. So that suddenly arrived without much notice, so there was lots of moving of furniture. But he's a lot more comfortable.

Two days after my brother's wedding the GP and palliative nurse did a joint visit, and they talked to us about anticipatory medicines. So in the event that sickness might be uncontrollable or Dad gets really agitated there are four particular medicines that can be just kept at home and administered by syringe by the district nurses. They're there if they're needed. So we had the conversation about that and those were requested. Our local pharmacist is also a family friend. They literally are in the next shop to Dad's shop, so they come and tell my youngest brother, who's now running Dad's business for him, about these and help him understand the point at which they might be needed. So we're getting a lot of really helpful advice.

First week of August, Dad has a fall in the bathroom because of the low blood pressure, and it knocks his confidence, so he's not venturing downstairs at all now. He wants to stay upstairs. And we're trying to encourage him as much as possible. He loved his walks in the garden. Mum and Dad have got a really nice garden. But he was having none of it. He wanted to stay upstairs.

Coming up to the August bank holiday, Dad's not coming downstairs now. He's had a couple more falls, and he's sleeping a lot more. Hospice are providing a night-sitting service, which is fantastic, because Mum is now sleeping in the same room as Dad and had been probably since about the middle of July, just so that she's nearby if he needs anything. And she refuses to let me share that burden with her.

It's probably three or four times a week, depending on the need of others that they're looking after as well. And the night-sitters are so caring and kind. Yet again Dad is making sure that they're okay. There was one evening in particular and this lovely sitter turned up and Dad said, oh, we've got a chair in the corner, nice comfy chair, you make sure you're comfortable, would you like a tea or coffee, we've got some doughnuts downstairs, would you like a doughnut? And we're like, who's looking after who here? That was just Dad. He just wanted to make sure that everybody else was looked after.

It was around August bank holiday that we decided actually that we might need the anticipatory medicines. The first injection just completely wipes him out for nearly forty-eight hours.

My dad was one of eight, and my mum's one of four. We've had a few visitors over the bank holiday and they've seen how poorly Dad is, and actually he's getting worse. And my aunt in the States wants to Facetime to see Dad. My dad has never liked Facetime. This request comes through my aunt in Solihull. I say no to her, and she says, well, we'll see what your brothers and your mum and dad think. I said, fine, have the conversation. And this was before the GP comes to visit. The GP comes to visit and we have a private conversation with her, myself, my brother and Mum, and we tell her how stressful it is. At this point there's lots of family round constantly and it's very difficult to focus on Dad. My other brother isn't helping. He is taking daily calls from my aunt and uncle in the States and insisting that they speak to Dad and waking Dad up when he's asleep and it's just not helping in the slightest.

The GP said, well, would you like me to go downstairs and talk to them? So the GP comes downstairs and she has a very blunt conversation with some of the family who were there that basically goes along the lines of: these are the last days of his life, this is the time where his immediate family should be spending that valuable time with him. She talks about this Facetime request and says that's utter nonsense. She says that immediate family are going to need a lot of support so the best thing you can do is support, and she points to me and my brother and his wife, support these three and his wife who's upstairs in a very upset state because we don't know what the next few days are going to bring. And actually it was very brave of her to do that, but also because she was the GP, she was independent, she was professional, that message carried authority …

So he's now got a syringe driver and that's administering morphine and other medication to him, and the nurses are coming and monitoring that. As we get to 31 August it's my mum and dad's forty-fourth wedding anniversary. It's a Saturday. We had lots of people in the day, and it's probably about eight o'clock. We've had a night-sitter the night before. They're very good at handing over to the district nurses as well, so they document everything in the yellow folder that's kept in Dad's room, but they also talk to each other as well. So that's fantastic because when somebody arrives you don't have to go over everything.

The evening district nurse comes and my brother and his wife go upstairs and are with Dad whilst she's just making him comfortable, and she says that she's not sure that she'll see us tomorrow because she's not sure that Dad will make it. And we just sit by Dad. The night-sitter comes in and she can see that it's very near the end. And Dad passes away about quarter past eleven that night. On his wedding anniversary. Surrounded by his family and all of our love and all that positivity to take him where he's going to.

The night that Dad passes, the night-sitter's fantastic: she phones the district nurses, they come in and remove the syringe driver, and then she makes Dad comfortable and just makes him look really presentable, and then gives us a little bit of time. She calls the 111 service, because we're in the middle of the night now, and we have to wait for a doctor to come and certify the death. So whilst we're waiting we've got some time to spend with Dad, and that was really important for us to do.

Then myself and my two brothers went to see the GP on Monday because the family GP had seen him within fourteen days, so we need that GP to sign the documentation. Unfortunately she's on holiday that day so we see somebody else. But actually that's quite smooth, and all the registration is absolutely fine. The district nurse who came on the Saturday evening and said, I don't think I'll see you, comes the day after to collect the paperwork, the yellow folder, because actually that's the NHS's property, and she's very sympathetic. It was actually quite nice to see her to thank her and all of her team.

We do have to wait for the hospital bed to be collected, and that seems to take an age. And I don't mind that so much, but my sister-in-law doesn't like the fact that that bed is in the room. She doesn't like it at all. But I can deal with that, I'm fine with that. There is a lot of phoning people, and this is where my practical head switches on and I'm doing all of this. In the meantime we have a lot of family come to visit us. The process of grieving is quite interesting in that it's now an open house, so people can literally turn up whenever they like to pay their respects. In one way that's open, but in another way it gives us no privacy at all. So for two solid weeks until Dad's funeral we have people, night in, night out, and my mum is exhausted, and there is no chance for a lie-in for her. There's no chance of any time for her at all to process what's happened, to even start to grieve, because culturally it's the norm. It's what happens.

And there were other bizarre rituals that are done, some of which I understand, others of which have no logic or rationale in terms of explanation, so I question them, and I get told that this is just how it is. Well, that's not good enough for me. Well, it's still going to happen because that's how it is. This isn't my mother saying it, this is other people saying that.

For example, because my father has passed away, after the crematorium service we go back to the temple and there is this little ceremony where my brother is given a turban as a way of acknowledging that he is now head of the household, and with that comes the responsibility of looking after the family. Well, he doesn't deserve that, quite frankly. And I question why it's given to the eldest son, not the eldest child. Well, you're a girl, what are you going to do with a turban? Well then, let's not do the ceremony. No, no, we've got to do it. Well, what would happen if you had no male siblings? Well, you wouldn't do it. Well then, let's not do it. No, no, it's got to be done. So this nonsense ceremony is done which means nothing to me or my younger brother.

OLDER AGE AND END OF LIFE: REFLECTIONS AND RESPONSES TO THESE STORIES

Immediate questions

1. Why is it important to take account of family circumstances in organising complex care for older people?
2. What may have been the reasons for some of the different responses of the statutory agencies to Rabiya's and James's situation – both of whom were looking after mothers with dementia?

3. How important do you think was the role that Kauri played in collaborating with healthcare professionals to organise her dad's care?
4. "Sometimes I go to appointments with Mum in my work clothes with my NHS lanyard on because I think I will be taken more seriously." Why does Rabiya think that is necessary?
5. James is disappointed with the dismissive way in which his mother's diagnosis is delivered. "It was a case of, right, there's your diagnosis … come back in twelve months, and that's it." What would a better response have looked like?

Strategic questions
1. What does Rabiya's story tell us about the intersection between racism and ageism in the NHS?
2. These stories have several examples of people "battling" the system to get better care for their loved ones. What are the wider implications of a system that needs to be "battled"?
3. What part can health and social care agencies play in managing family tensions and differences during serious illness and at the end of life?
4. These stories contain a number of examples of really good care and professional practice. What makes them good?

REFERENCES

Age UK (2019) *Improving Healthcare (England)*, Age UK, May, www.ageuk.org.uk/globalassets/age-uk/documents/policy-positions/care-and-support/age-uk-improving-healthcare-policy-position.pdf (accessed 28 March 2021).

Mid Staffordshire NHS Foundation Trust Public Inquiry (2013) *Report of the Mid Staffordshire NHS Foundation Trust Public Inquiry: Executive summary*, HC 947 (London: Stationery Office), www.midstaffspublicinquiry.com/sites/default/files/report/Executive%20summary.pdf (accessed 3 January 2021).

Nasim, A. (2014) "The demise of the Liverpool Care Pathway", *GM*, www.gmjournal.co.uk/the-demise-of-the-liverpool-care-pathway (accessed 3 January 2021).

NHS (2020) "About dementia: dementia guide", www.nhs.uk/conditions/dementia/about (accessed 3 January 2021).

Oliver, D. (2015) "Leading change in diagnosis and support for people living with dementia", blog post, King's Fund, 3 February, www.kingsfund. org.uk/blog/2015/02/leading-change-diagnosis-and-support-people-living-dementia (accessed 3 January 2021).

WHO (2015) *World Report on Ageing and Health 2015* (Geneva: WHO) http://who.int/ageing/publications/world-report-2015/en/ (accessed 3 January 2021).

❧ 8 ❧

CONCLUSION

CHAPTER SUMMARY

In Chapter 1 we introduced Osler's injunction – "Just listen to your patient, he is telling you the diagnosis". In this conclusion we examine how far Osler is heeded in today's NHS. We assess the value of gathering stories in this way as a contribution to truly listening to patients and their families. We reflect on the extent to which the spirit of the NHS Constitution is being upheld.

From the stories we identify five dimensions of care which is organised around patients: kindness, attentiveness, empowerment, organisational competence and professional competence. We compare these themes with the case and evidence for patient-centred care outlined in Chapter 1. We consider what the stories tell us about the things that patients value, the extent to which these things are put into practice, and what the obstacles are. We reflect on the five themes as the basis for a call to action for improvement. We discuss vital questions of context: in particular, straitened funding and workforce shortages in the NHS, and the experiences of COVID-19. Finally we touch on future trends, for example the rise of digital healthcare, and consider the implications for better organising care around patients. After this chapter there is a list of further resources that readers might find useful.

LISTENING TO PATIENTS

As the compilers of this book, we have been privileged to hear these stories. The experience has been hugely rewarding, and hard. We sometimes felt strong emotional responses, to the point of tears, not only on a first hearing or reading, but also in the subsequent editing process. Listening required emotional labour.

In reality we had it easy. We had plenty of time and good conditions for listening. We were unencumbered by any associated requirement to take action. It is very different for healthcare professionals who have to listen in busy, hectic and sometimes stressful circumstances. They may lack time, there might be shortages of staff and equipment, they might have to work with poor systems and processes. They might have their own personal difficulties. No wonder cursory questioning and inattentiveness can take place instead of deep listening.

The stories also suggest a deeper problem: that in parts of the NHS there are professional and organisational cultures that don't allow for patients' concerns to be heard. The Cumberlege Review into the safety of certain medicines and medical devices, published in July 2020, just a month after we obtained our last story, makes sobering reading in this regard. This inquiry heard accounts from more than 700 patients, mainly women, who have suffered harm, over decades, as a result of – or compounded by – not being listened to. They tell of severe damage to their unborn babies as a result of being given a pregnancy test drug, or epilepsy medication. Others relate experiences of how the surgical insertion of a vaginal mesh has caused awful pain and incontinence, and turned their lives upside down forever. The chair of the inquiry, Baroness Julia Cumberlege, talks of taking these stories to her grave (IMMD Safety Review, 2020).

GENERAL THEMES

The picture provided by the Care Quality Commission State of Health Care Report of 2019/20 (CQC, 2020) mentioned in Chapter 1 is consistent with the general tenor of these stories. While most care is good, poor experiences centre on difficulty in access to care, services not working in a joined-up way, people having to "chase" to get the care they need, problems with information and communication, and the caring burden for families.

So this book confirms that there is some way to go before we can say that the principles of the NHS Constitution are being consistently upheld:

> The NHS belongs to the people. It is there to improve our health and wellbeing, supporting us to keep mentally and physically well, to get

better when we are ill and, when we cannot fully recover, to stay as
well as we can to the end of our lives. It works at the limits of science
– bringing the highest levels of human knowledge and skill to save
lives and improve health. It touches our lives at times of basic human
need, when care and compassion are what matter most. (Department
of Health and Social Care, 2021: 1)

The Constitution emphasises the centrality of professional competence, holistic care and kindness. Similar themes emerge from the
stories we heard. We have identified five themes which, for us, sum up
the difference that well-organised care makes to patients. In accordance
with the spirit of this book, we offer them as an insight, a provocation
and a call to action, rather than as a definitive judgement. These themes
are depicted in figures 8.1 and 8.2 below, as we see them as intercon-
nected, and also as pillars in a house.

The first theme is **kindness.** In the stories, professionals demonstrated kindness when they kept their promises, believed their patients,
were generous with their time, rang them at home, conveyed warmth
and refused to give up on them and their problems. Kind professionals were "on the side" of our storytellers and not judgemental. They
understood the impact of delays in diagnosis and wrong diagnoses. After
a difficult time securing care for her mum with early-onset dementia
(see Chapter 7, Story 22), **Rabiya** found a physiotherapist who was the
epitome of kindness:

> Her name is Lily. I won't forget her name because she was such an amazing
> person … [My mum's] in a lot of pain and Lily just got it. I didn't have to
> justify what I was saying. She just understood. She just listened to me and
> she said, I understand. I remember she got a walking stick out and it was one
> of those hospital walking sticks, the grey ones, and my mum looked at it and
> she said, I'm not having that old woman stick. She was obviously saying it in
> Bengali to me. I was like, oh, gosh, how can I say to Lily that she doesn't want
> that stick? I'm really sorry, Lily, I know this is going to sound really childish
> but her previous stick was black, can she get a black stick? Lily was like, oh, yes
> … I completely understand, yes, no worries. If she thinks it's an old woman's
> stick, that's completely understandable … and she was just so supportive …
> She just went and got the black stick. Mum then was quite happy with that and
> she responded well, so when Lily was doing some of the exercises with her she
> was laughing along with Mum, engaging with her. Mum didn't understand
> what she was saying but Mum could tell from her body language she was being
> supportive and she just responded really well and it put me at ease as well.

Casual instances of unkindness and thoughtlessness can be so hurtful:

> *Jim had a hernia when he was quite small. We went into the room and the doctor that was going to do it asked if he could bring some students in and I said yes. And then they took Jim's pad off and he said to them, "You've never seen anything like this before and you never will again."* (Lucinda, the mother of **Jim**, Chapter 3, Story 4)

> *Eventually I left my GP when he told me that I needed to stop trying to get better because this is obviously what God wants for me.* (**Venetia**, Chapter 4, Story 11)

The second theme is **attentiveness.** Above all, this is about listening and observing closely, and the importance of focussing on the person as well as on the illness. It might include keeping an open mind about diagnosis. The stories indicate the importance of picking up cues, knowing when "labelling" can be helpful, as well as problematic, when patients would prefer a relaxed or a more formal style of communication, and when there might be mixed messages and dissent among family members, particularly when the illness is serious.

Attentiveness underpins an effective therapeutic relationship. In **Kauri**'s story in Chapter 7 (Story 25) the family GP understood what was going on and was able to help when tensions in the family were rising as Kauri's father neared his death:

> *The GP comes to visit and we have a private conversation with her ... and we tell her how stressful it is. At this point there's lots of family round constantly and it's very difficult to focus on Dad. My other brother isn't helping. He is taking daily calls from my aunt and uncle in the States and insisting that they speak to Dad and waking Dad up when he's asleep. ...*
> *The GP said, well, would you like me to go downstairs and talk to them? So... she has a very blunt conversation ... that basically goes along the lines of: these are the last days of his life, this is the time where his immediate family should be spending that valuable time with him ... [They] are going to need a lot of support so the best thing you can do is ... and she points to me and my brother and his wife, support these three and his wife who's upstairs in a very upset state because we don't know what the next few days are going to bring. And actually it was very brave of her to do that, but also because she was the GP, she was independent, she was professional, that message carried authority.*

The third theme is **empowerment**. In Chapter 1 we discussed the contested terminology concerning patient-centred care. The term "empowerment" also has both its supporters and detractors. Some activists and campaigners detect a whiff of paternalism in the notion that a professional should empower them, as in: "I already have power, thank you very much, I don't need your authority to exert it". Others react to the individualism embedded in the concept, pointing out that inequalities of power – for example, relating to social class, ethnicity and gender – are structural, requiring collective solutions beyond the realm of the citizen–professional or patient–clinician relationship (McLaughlin, 2015). These considerations can lead to the search for alternative formulations such as "power-sharing", "working collaboratively" etc. For the purposes of this book, we prefer to stick with the relative elegance and simplicity of "empowerment", while recognising that the term is not without problems.

There is often a power imbalance between the professional and the patient. In these stories, that appears to be particularly true when the professional is a doctor, rather than a nurse, therapist or emergency staff. A key determinant of the power imbalance is information asymmetry. The clinician has technical knowledge, expertise and practical experience that the patient cannot match. On the other hand, the patient has expertise and knowledge about their life and about living with particular conditions. So who is actually the expert here? As **Joanna** puts it (Chapter 4, Story 9):

> One of the GPs that I've chosen not to see actually has a mug on his top shelf that says, don't confuse my seven years at med school with your Google search. Which … intelligent people find very offensive. Because, don't confuse your twenty-minute lecture at medical school on my condition with my fifty-seven years of living with it.

Professional power can be wielded to good effect, as in Kauri's story above. It also comes to the fore when the patient lacks agency. For example, when the patient is acutely ill, the relationship is necessarily less of a partnership, the professional takes charge and the critical ingredient for the patient is not agency but the trust which they have in the professional, making them feel safe and cared for.

Such cases apart, the normal requirement is for the professional to be sensitive to the patient's own expertise, intelligence and capacity, and their need for control, and to adapt their style accordingly. This is particularly important for supporting people to take control of their lifelong health conditions. Patients use the Internet to find further details of their conditions and to check the doctor's diagnosis. Many people with long-term conditions find self-help or peer support groups helpful to get more information about their condition, to track whether their experience of care is "normal", and to derive practical and emotional support. Some patients are able to access more formal self-management training and support programmes. The job of the professional is to go with the grain of such self-help efforts and help where they can. For some people there is a natural progression from gaining control of their conditions to becoming involved in supporting improvements in service organisation and delivery. Some of our storytellers had such experiences of patient participation, which have been important routes to personal development and empowerment.

Another important dimension of the power dynamic is that many people's experiences of ill health and of care are overlaid with bias, stigma and exclusion as a result of their condition, ethnicity, age or other characteristics. Some of our stories touch on these issues and the intersections between these areas of discrimination.

The fourth theme is **professional competence.** Many issues concerning technical professional competence – and variations in the clinical quality of care – are beyond the scope of this book. They relate to such matters as training, supervision and clinical governance. On the other hand it is clear from these stories that perceptions of competence are highly important for patients and linked to the other themes of patient-centredness. We were concerned at the frequency with which issues of professional competence arose in the stories, particularly in the context of mental health. **Jonathan**, whose son **Dan** was seriously ill and hospitalised with a physical illness for three weeks (see Chapter 3, Story 3), had some concerns about the clinical competence of the ward nurses, despite their evident compassion:

> I can't think of a nurse who wasn't kind and caring. But they weren't always good at the basics.

An important strand of professional competence is personal conduct. Patients are highly sensitive to aspects such as reliability and good time management, and the absence of these is keenly felt. These aspects of personal conduct can also be considered part of professionalism – behaviours that are both important in themselves and as signals to patients and families of trustworthiness.

Delays in diagnosis are distressing for patients for obvious reasons. This is a fraught area of care because diagnosis always carries an element of uncertainty, and the diagnosis of rare conditions can be especially difficult. A misdiagnosis is not always an example of incompetence. GPs are generalists who cannot be expert in all conditions. Nor can they refer every worried patient to a specialist. Indeed, their referral activity is generally highly constrained by local commissioners on cost grounds.

What, therefore, can patients reasonably expect? On the basis of the stories in this book, we have to go back to Osler: listen to your patient because he is telling you the diagnosis. A common theme of some of the stories was the feeling of not being listened to, when the storyteller as the patient knew that something was wrong. Clinicians have to listen and keep an open mind. They must recognise the limits of their expertise and where necessary – and within organisational and system constraints – seek help from other experts. In the light of new information, they have to be willing to acknowledge that an initial diagnosis was wrong and to change their mind. Patients can be surprisingly forgiving of errors made in good faith. It is harder to forgive professional arrogance, stubbornness and defensiveness. Meanwhile, referral systems need to be flexible and should not override clinical judgement.

The final theme is **organisational competence**. The first four themes are very much to do with the abilities and personal qualities of individual healthcare professionals. But individual caregivers work in organisations and systems of care. The extent to which their personal kindness, attentiveness and other qualities can cut through and make a difference is influenced by the wider system: its efficiency, accessibility and responsiveness. In Chapter 3, discussing his son's care over a three-week period in hospital, **Jonathan** (Chapter 3, Story 3) described his confusion about who was in charge:

> It was actually quite difficult to work out what status and authority the different nurses had. I think there is a colour coding in the uniforms. It was never clear. There was never the equivalent of what the consultants did. They would tend to introduce themselves and say, "Hi, I'm a consultant this and I'm a consultant that and my name is so and so." Whereas the nurses would tend to introduce themselves by their first names and say, "Hi, I'm so and so and I'm on duty tonight," but it wasn't always clear how senior they were and how much authority they had. You want to know who's in charge.

Time is not just in the gift of the individual caregiver but also how systems such as outpatient clinic appointment timetables are constructed. **Shona** who had breast cancer (Chapter 5, Story 15) describes the impact of not being given much time:

> When you go there you've only got five minutes with them. It's only at the beginning when you are diagnosed that they seem to have more time. After two

or three years you're just a normal patient and they have to tick the boxes and in five minutes you're out the door.

These stories frequently tell of examples where the patient, or the carer, needed to "work the system" to coordinate the care when that was not being done by the system. As **Joanna** in Chapter 4 (Story 9) put it:

I've often said that some aspects of the NHS should be run by Ocado, because it is actually a logistics company.

Signposting is an important aspect of system competence, and a lack of this can cause patients, and carers in particular, to feel very alone, as expressed by **Sheila** in Chapter 7 (Story 24) while she was struggling to care for her husband with dementia:

Everything that I've discovered, I've discovered on my own. I didn't know who the gatekeepers were, the signposters. I now am aware that there are useful people but I often discovered them fairly randomly:, an article in the local paper offering some sort of carers' support … coffee meeting, for instance … which I attended and then found there were other resources that I could access via a very efficient carers' forum. It's all been really random.

Connected with signposting, fragmentation appears all too common, though it is not universal. Where care is well integrated, it makes a huge difference to patients and to their carers. GPs are well placed to be coordinators but don't appear always to rise to this task. This may reflect the limited capacity of primary care services, which have experienced big rises in demand in recent years, without the substantial funding increases that have gone into the hospital sector.

Organisational competence also includes providing, where possible, continuity of care to individuals. The service needs to be especially alert to the challenges faced by people with rare conditions, because many clinicians haven't come across their condition before. **Rabiya**'s account in Chapter 7 (Story 22) also underlines the challenge of providing services that accord with principles of equality, diversity and inclusion.

Figure 8.1 is an aid to consider the interconnectedness of these dimensions of patient-centred care. The stories suggest the importance of these linkages:

It's the clinical competence along with the compassion, and one without the other doesn't work – it has to be both together. And I think that's what is wrong with a lot of healthcare: people can be very proficient at one or the other and it's those two together. (**Cathy**, Chapter 2, Story 1)

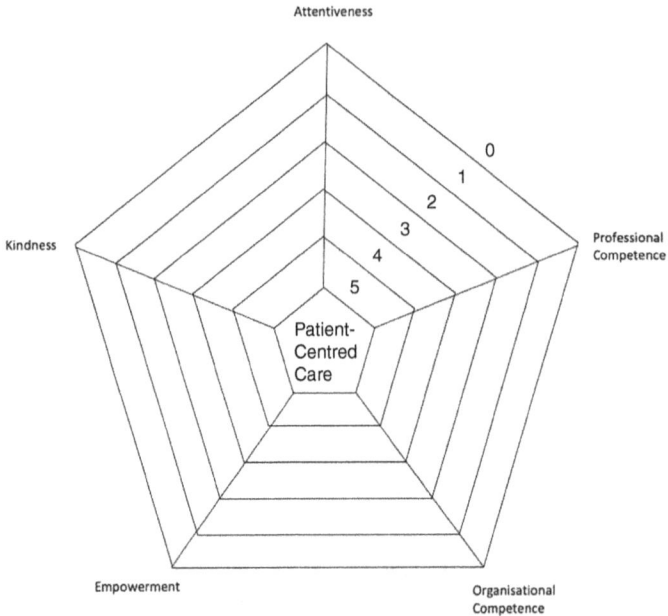

Figure 8.1   How well is the care organised around the patient?
5 = Excellent, 4 = Very Good, 3 = Good, 2 = Fair, 1 = Poor, 0 = Very Poor

The figure can be helpful for those of you who want to take a closer look at one or more of the stories in this book to analyse what is really going on. You can plot how well the care is organised along the five dimensions. Are there links between them? How hard is it to offer kindness in the absence of organisational competence, for example? For healthcare professionals and managers, the figure could also be helpful as a tool to reflect on patient stories that you yourselves seek out or have otherwise heard about – perhaps when responding to a complaint or a compliment, or participating in Schwartz rounds (opportunities for staff, from all disciplines, to come together in a safe space, to share experiences of caring for patients and the associated learning).

In a different way of organising the main themes, Figure 8.2 depicts them as five pillars which we suggest symbolise the solid foundations of care that is well organised around patients. We have deliberately left the pillars blank so that readers of these stories can themselves attribute adjectives that relate to the themes.

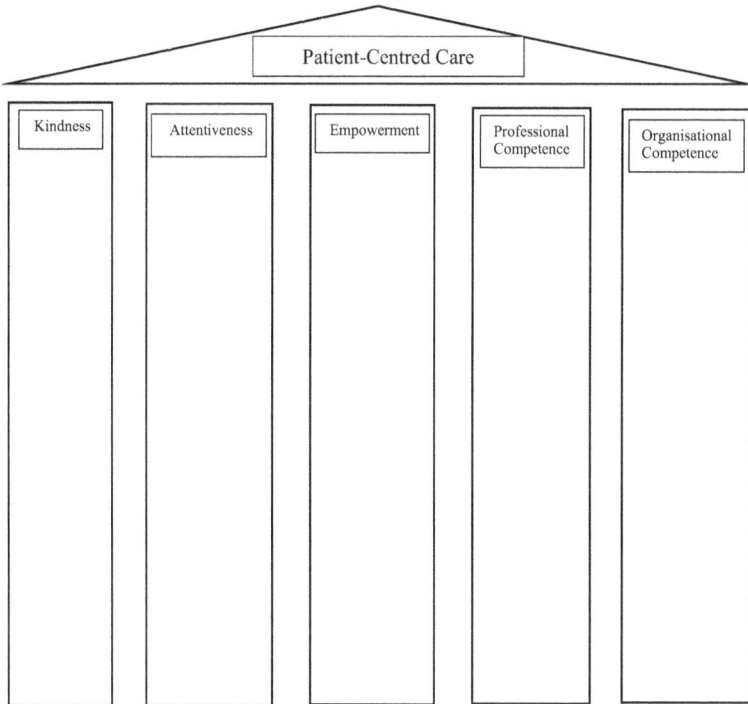

Figure 8.2 The five pillars of well-organised care around patients

IMPACT AND LEARNING

This book will have different meanings and impacts for different groups of readers. We hope that it will have broad relevance. For the general reader, we hope that the stories will offer new and useful insights. You may find some of the stories uplifting and others unexpectedly shocking or distressing, as they show the NHS at its very best, and also when it falls significantly short. The book is in not a "how-to" guide for navigating the complexities of the NHS, but the stories might help you think back on some past personal experiences and on how you might approach the NHS differently in future, in view of some its flaws illustrated by these stories. If you are a patient or carer currently "battling" with the system, we hope you derive some hope and encouragement from these stories.

For voluntary organisations, disease-specific charities and support groups, there is much here to pump up your tyres. The stories show the valuable complementary role of the voluntary sector in terms of providing information and peer support, and pointers for how closer working with the statutory healthcare organisations could be beneficial.

For politicians, policymakers and commentators, the book is a sharp reminder of how far the NHS has to go in order to make the values of the NHS Constitution a consistent day-in day-out reality. Policies, programmes, workforce strategies and funding arrangements need to do better to produce care that is consistently well organised around patients. As we enter the fourth industrial revolution, 5G and post-COVID-19 era, there is an opportunity to deconstruct and reconstruct services in a different way (see below).

For NHS leaders and managers, some of the stories will make for uncomfortable reading. To what extent could patients in your own hospital or community service be experiencing the kind of lack of attention described in some of these accounts? It is understandably easy to react defensively to evidence of poor care. This was all about workforce shortages and funding problems, you might say. Or, this sort of thing wouldn't happen on my watch. Others may see this as an opportunity to kick-start a fresh conversation with staff and with patients in their care – how are we doing and how can we do better? How can we improve the experience of care for people from Black, Asian and other minority ethnic backgrounds?

For healthcare professionals, especially doctors, at whom some of the harshest criticism has been directed, an immediate defensive reaction to some of the negative experiences described by patients may be natural. How can we provide the care we would like to, with all the deficiencies of the system we are working in? How can we ever measure up to Google? We hope that, going beyond that first instinctive response, reading the stories will yield creative ideas for improving services. In addition to the versatility and creativity shown during the COVID-19 pandemic, clinicians from all disciplines have already demonstrated how versatile and clever they are at this in the quality-improvement work that has been going on quietly in parts of the NHS for over a decade now, often working closely with patients as a starting point.

FUTURE PROSPECTS

In the Introduction to this book we outlined some of the limitations of our approach. This is a small collection of stories. Many voices are absent. We have not, for example, listened directly to a child, or a patient hospitalised with COVID-19, or a care home resident. All their stories, and others, deserve to be told, documented and acknowledged in order to understand fully how to organise care around patients. We hope that others will pick up the baton. But we think there is already enough material here, and from other sources, to stimulate a call to action to reset a sense of purpose, priorities and professionalism for patient-centred care. Current circumstances present a unique moment in which this can be done.

COVID-19 has been a "stop" moment for the NHS in 2020 and 2021. On the one hand, normal services have been suspended, and waits for diagnosis and treatment are longer than ever. Many health and care staff have lost their lives as a result of the infection. Staff burnout is a serious concern. There is the potential for vulnerable patients to feel more stranded than ever. **Jonathan**'s story about the emergency care of his acutely ill son **Dan** (Chapter 3, Story 3) is a case in point. Dan spent three weeks on a paediatric ward in a London hospital at the height of the pandemic. His parents reported a sense that, as in wartime, the only nurses left behind on the (non-COVID) hospital ward were very young staff still in training, or a few very senior experienced staff, perhaps too old to be deployed on the COVID-19 frontline.

On the other hand, something has happened in the NHS which is similar to Schumpeter's notion of creative destruction, derived from economic theory. COVID-19 has prompted instantaneous revolutions in processes from within, simultaneously destroying old practices and creating new ones. Clinicians from all disciplines in GP practices, hospitals and in community services have moved swiftly to telephone or online consultations and to remote prescribing. The days of standard hospital outpatient follow-up appointments of questionable value (for example, as described by **Robert** in Chapter 7, Story 21) may suddenly be over. New hospitals usually take ten years from first design to the day of opening – pop-up hospital wards have been built in a fortnight.

5G offers the opportunity to embed the digitisation of the NHS, a move which has accelerated with the advent of the COVID-19 pandemic. Technology is a cornerstone of the future of healthcare, and the NHS Long Term Plan is predicated on the rise and adoption of digital services and data sharing. 5G will allow diagnoses using artificial intelligence (AI), enable remote monitoring of the millions of people with long-term conditions, and facilitate remote access to specialist consultations and advice.

Designing digitised care systems around the needs of patients rather than around the needs of organisations and professionals will remain a challenge. Those who are at least partially digitally excluded cannot be left behind in this brave new world. Concerns about data security will have to be addressed. Above all, it will be important to build into the design the right ways of working, with the necessary attitudes and behaviours. However much the technology advances, healthcare will remain a fundamentally human endeavour. Kindness, attentiveness, patient empowerment, professional and organisational competence will all still matter.

REFERENCES

CQC (2020) *The State of Health Care and Adult Social Care in England 2019/20*, HC 799 (Newcastle: CQC), www.cqc.org.uk/sites/default/files/20201016_stateofcare1920_fullreport.pdf (accessed 3 January 2021).

Department of Health and Social Care (2021) NHS Constitution for England www.gov.uk/government/publications/the-nhs-constitution-for-england/the-nhs-constitution-for-england (accessed 28 March 2021)

IMMD Safety Review (2020) *First Do No Harm: The report of the Independent Medicines and Medical Devices Safety Review* (Cumberlege Report) (London: IMMD Safety Review), www.immdsreview.org.uk/downloads/IMMDSReview_web.pdf (accessed 3 January 2021).

McLaughlin, K. (2015) *Empowerment: A critique* (London: Routledge).

FURTHER PRACTICAL RESOURCES

THIS.Institute, **"Not quite right"** (https://info.thisinstitute.cam.ac.uk/ not-quite-right)
This is a video which is a scenario about a patient who has a stroke. It's played by actors: it focusses on how care can be better organised and the need for research-driven improvements.

NHS England, "The House of Care" (www.england.nhs.uk/ourwork/ clinical-policy/ltc/house-of-care/)
The House of Care model is a framework for care for people living with long-term conditions. It recognises the need for care coordination, emotional and psychological support, predictive rather than reactive services, and multiple comorbidities becoming the norm.

Care Opinion (www.careopinion.org.uk)
Care Opinion is a place where people can share their experience of health or care services. As of July 2020, over 500 organisations were using Care Opinion to listen to what patients, service users and carers are saying. Care Opinion works with health and care providers, commissioners, health boards, regulators, professional bodies, educators, researchers and patient groups.

Point of Care Foundation (www.pointofcarefoundation.org.uk)
The Point of Care Foundation works to improve patients' experience of care and to increase support for the staff who work with them. The website contains useful tools (for example, how to use patient experiences for improving services), impactful videos of patient stories and Schwartz rounds, where staff explore honestly and openly instances where care has not been as good as they would have liked to provide.

Healthtalk (www.healthtalk.org)
Healthtalk provides thousands of videos of patient experiences with lots of different health conditions to help people to understand and prepare for what lies ahead.

Patient Experience Library (www.patientlibrary.net/cgi-bin/library.cgi)
The Patient Experience Library provides a patient experience research and evidence database.

Patient Voices (www.patientvoices.org.uk)
Patient Voices use stories to help patients understand their conditions.

APPENDIX:
ANONYMISED LIST OF INTERVIEWEES AND BACKGROUND DETAILS

Name	Principal health issue(s) discussed	Background (gender, age, equality group, social education or status)	Interview with (and date)	Key issues
Chapter 2: Pregnancy and childbirth				
Cathy	Recently gave birth	Female, 30s White English Healthcare professional	Jeremy February 2020	Very difficult birth, mostly well handled, with a few lapses in care; some reflections on what constitutes good maternity care; implications for professional practice.
James	Carer for mum with dementia and now new dad	Male, 50s White English Secondary education, professional	Naomi February 2020	As new dad, positive experiences of being included by maternity staff. Trauma of birth for his partner not well handled by NHS.
Chapter 3: Children and young people				
Dan	Teenage boy. Story told by dad, Jonathan	Male, 16 White British Middle-class professional background	Naomi June 2020	Experience of hospitalisation for acute illness during the COVID-19 pandemic.

Name	Principal health issue(s) discussed	Background (gender, age, equality group, social education or status)	Interview with (and date)	Key issues
Jim	Young man living with severe disabilities who died aged 36. Story told by parents Justin and Lucinda	Male, from birth to 36 White English Middle-class professional background	Naomi June 2020	Difficulties of caring for a young man with serious disabilities.
Eve	Remembering a childhood diagnosis of type 1 diabetes	Female	Naomi January 2018	
Finbar	Scoliosis. Story told by parent Eileen	Male, teenager Middle-class background	Naomi December 2019	Length of time to get to see specialist consultant in tertiary facility. GP (and mum) knew diagnosis but they still had to go through hospital consultant for onward referral. Mum tracked and chivvied tertiary unit for appointments and to make sure operation was scheduled. Experience of support group very helpful.

Name	Principal health issue(s) discussed	Background (gender, age, equality group, social education or status)	Interview with (and date)	Key issues
Chapter 4: Managing a long-term health condition as an adult				
Katie	Diabetes, other conditions	Female, 50s White English Secondary education. Not able to work	Naomi April 2018	Ups and downs of getting good care for type 1 diabetes and complications. Postcode lottery battle to get continuous testing device on the NHS. Kindness of some of the GPs at the practice – also not having to repeat oneself. Very difficult to access mental health support to tackle the psychological impact of this long-term condition; husband has never been offered support as a carer.
Tim	Epilepsy	Male, 30s White English Middle-class background	Jeremy January 2020	Difficulty of living with epilepsy; stigma; drugs balancing act; importance of family and friends; great nurses and paramedics; good and bad doctor experiences; difficulty of finding a good specialist; pros and cons of support groups: "I am more than epilepsy".

Name	Principal health issue(s) discussed	Background (gender, age, equality group, social education or status)	Interview with (and date)	Key issues
Joanna	Various long-term conditions, including rare condition. Also parent carer of child with long-term conditions	Female, adult White English Professional	Jeremy January 2020	High-handed doctors; difficulty of getting diagnosis; fragmentation of care; poor basic administration; difficulty of getting improvements without formal complaints.
Jasmin	Lupus	Female, 30s BAME Middle-class	Jeremy February 2020	Four years to get a diagnosis of lupus; "I knew something was wrong. I wasn't listened to"; private doctors got to the bottom of the problem; "my whole body was shutting down"; pros and cons of belonging to a support group; poor experience of NHS physiotherapy; generally having to battle.
Venetia	Chronic fatigue syndrome	Female, late 20s White English University degree. Works in admin	Naomi June 2017	Lack of support for the condition, particularly from GP; pros and cons of support group; having to search oneself to understand the condition; lack of local clinical service.

Name	Principal health issue(s) discussed	Background (gender, age, equality group, social education or status)	Interview with (and date)	Key issues
Chapter 5: Adult acute care and cancer				
Jill	Accident – dislocated knee	Female, 50s White English Professional, former teacher	Jeremy January 2020	Waiting for an ambulance; pain; great nurses; brusque doctors; successful rehab but had to fight for it; poor organisation of wound care.
Andrea	Surgery – gallbladder operation	Female, older White English Left school at 16. Manual work in hotel industry	Naomi December 2019	Successful outcome; pleased with lack of waiting; care seemed to be well coordinated; surprised to be treated in a private hospital as an NHS patient.
Lucy	Sepsis	Female, older White English Retired healthcare professional	Naomi April 2018	Hospitalised with sepsis; experience of different quality of care and treatment on different wards; problem with accessing medical records between hospitals; patient lives with severe and enduring mental illness.
Shona	Breast cancer	Female, 40s BAME	Jeremy June 2020	Experiences of being diagnosed with breast cancer; treatment and of living as a cancer survivor.

Name	Principal health issue(s) discussed	Background (gender, age, equality group, social education or status)	Interview with (and date)	Key issues
Chapter 6: Mental health and mental illness				
Audrey	Family member of mental health service user	Female, 30s White English Healthcare professional	Naomi December 2016	Length of time to get diagnosis of severe mental health problem for family member.
Stanley	Mental health – bipolar disorder	Male, 40s Black African	Jeremy December 2019	The importance of seeing the person; the importance of work to mental health; stigma.
Alan	Mental health – bipolar disorder	Male, 40s White English University degree	Jeremy December 2019	Continuity of care; therapeutic relationship; poorly designed services; patient participation as a route to personal development.
Nathan	Mental health	Male, teenager White, English, gay	Jeremy January 2020	Human qualities of the therapist; continuity of care; being believed; impact of diagnosis/misdiagnosis; labelling; importance of NHS/school liaison; importance of good receptionists.
Lucy	Lifelong severe and enduring mental illness	Female, older White English Retired healthcare professional	Naomi April 2018	Lack of communication between hospital and primary care for mental health problems.

Name	Principal health issue(s) discussed	Background (gender, age, equality group, social education or status)	Interview with (and date)	Key issues
Chapter 7: Older age and end of life				
Robert	Bowel and heart problems	Male, 80s White English University degree, retired manager	Naomi January 2020	Involved in patient participation after retirement; various illnesses, including stomach problem, heart attack and joint problems; fragmentation in the NHS; lack of clarity on role of district/community nurse.
Rabiya	Carer of mum with dementia	Female, 30s Muslim Asian University degree, professional	Naomi February 2020	Struggles with getting diagnosis for mum; experiences of discrimination; poor support from general practice and other parts of NHS and social care; one episode of real kindness from a physio.
James	Carer for mum with dementia and now new dad	Male, 50s White English Secondary education, professional	Naomi February 2020	Looked after mum for many years, put life on hold to do this; issues and good and bad stories; patient participation, particularly around needs of carers.

Name	Principal health issue(s) discussed	Background (gender, age, equality group, social education or status)	Interview with (and date)	Key issues
Sheila	Wife of man with a diagnosis of dementia	Female, 60s White English University degree, retired professional	Naomi December 2017	Difficulty in getting diagnosis; battle to get care in place; poor experiences of GP practice.
Kauri	Carer of dad who had pancreatic cancer	Female, 40s Sikh Asian University degree, professional	Naomi February 2020	Many episodes of excellent care and support from hospital and GP; delay in diagnosis; three-month hospital stay; end-of-life care supported by district nurses, visiting hospice staff and GP; challenge from managing the wider family.

INDEX

EU authorised representative for GPSR:
Easy Access System Europe, Mustamäe tee 50,
10621 Tallinn, Estonia
gpsr.requests@easproject.com